Clinical Examination in Orthopedics

K Mohan Iyer

Clinical Examination
in Orthopedics

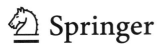 Springer

K Mohan Iyer
Consultant Orthopedic Surgeon
Bangalore
Karnataka State
India

ISBN 978-0-85729-970-3   e-ISBN 978-0-85729-971-0
DOI 10.1007/978-0-85729-971-0
Springer London Dordrecht Heidelberg New York

British Library Cataloguing in Publication Data
A catalogue record for this book is available from the British Library

Library of Congress Control Number: 2011940457

Printed on acid-free paper

Springer is part of Springer Science+Business Media (www.springer.com)

Dedicated to my wife, Nalini K Mohan
And
Daughter, Dr. Deepa Iyer
And
Son, Mr. Rohit Iyer

Foreword

It gives me immense pleasure to write this foreword for my dear friend Dr. K Mohan Iyer for his book *Clinical Examination in Orthopedics*. This book has been written step-wise, enumerating various aspects of the importance of clinical examination derived by laying one's hands on the affected parts. A thorough clinical examination can help us to arrive at a tentative differential diagnosis of the condition and hence help in investigations with numerous further tests which are relevant to the given condition. Handling a given case in this way is far more important than the diagnosis of the condition, and this comes with practicing the same approach many times. Learning this is essential for anyone embarking on a career in orthopedics.

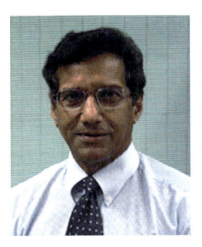

Singapore

Prof. Shamal Das De, M.Ch. Orth. Liv., M.B.B.S. Calc.,
F.R.C.S. (Ed), F.R.C.S. (Orth.) Ed, F.R.C.S.,
AM Sing., M.D. NUS.

Preface

This book has been written after many years of working in orthopedics at four well-recognized universities in different parts of the world: namely, Bombay University, Liverpool University, London University, and Bangalore University. I have had the pleasure of working in various capacities in these universities and would expect any candidate (whether undergraduate or postgraduate) to know these fundamental basic examination criteria when arriving at the various features of discussion, which are extremely important in getting good marks in their final examinations. This book outlines the basic points which must be kept in mind when examining any bone or joint in orthopedics.

I would like to thank my dear friend and colleague Dilip Malhotra, M.S. Orth., M.Ch. Orth., F.I.C.S., senior consultant orthopedic surgeon, International Hospital of Bahrain, Bahrain, for his timely and valuable help with the X-rays and photographs for this book, without which it would have been very difficult for me to complete this book. I would also like to thank my other colleagues, in particular Dushyant H. Thakkar, M.S. Orth., M.Ch. Orth., F.R.C.S. Orth., senior consultant orthopedic surgeon, London, UK, who has also given me X-rays and photographs for this book. Above all, it gives me great pleasure to thank immensely my respected teacher, L.N. Vora, M.S. (Bom.), F.C.P.S. (Bom.), F.R.C.S. (Eng.), M.Ch. Orth. (L'Pool), Hon. Orthopedic Surgeon, Sir. H. N. Hospital, Mumbai; Hon. Prof. of Orthopedics (Retd.), Seth G. S. Medical College, Mumbai; Hon. Orthopedic Surgeon (Retd.) K.E.M. Hospital, Mumbai; for his kind permission to insert the entire chapter "Examination of Gait" in my book. Finally I would like to express my sincere thanks to Mr. Steffan D. Clements, editor, Clinical Medicine, Springer (London), for his guidance in the preparation of this book.

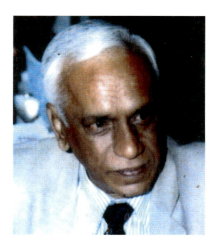

Karnataka, India   K Mohan Iyer, M.Ch. Orth. (Liverpool, UK),
                                           M.S. Orth. (Bom), F.C.P.S. Orth. (Bom),
                                           D'Orth. (Bom), M.B.B.S. (Bom).

Contents

Chapter 1
Examination for Diseases of the Bone

A bony lesion or a swelling of the bone is always fixed to it and cannot be moved away from the bone.

Completion of a case history should clarify certain informative points:

1. *Age*: A solitary cyst of the bone is seen in children, after which it becomes rare. Osteogenesis imperfecta (brittle bones) usually presents with multiple fractures, dwarfism, and deformities since birth. Acute osteomyelitis is seen commonly in children, whereas tuberculous osteomyelitis may be seen at any age. Nearly all benign bone tumors occur in adolescents and at younger ages, whereas primary malignant bone tumors mainly occur in young people, and secondary carcinoma of bone is usually seen in those older than 40 years of age.

2. *Onset and progression*: A history of trauma is usually obtained in acute osteomyelitis and osteosarcoma. Spontaneous development of swelling is mainly seen in cases of bone tumors. An acute onset with a high rise of temperature is usually seen in acute osteomyelitis. A gradual insidious onset is normally seen in chronic osteomyelitis. Malignant tumors grow very rapidly, and the history is relatively short once the patient has discovered the swelling.

3. *Pain*: Pain is normally associated with inflammation, but in certain cases of osteosarcoma, pain comes first followed by swelling later on. One must note the character of the pain – whether it is throbbing, which is usually seen in inflammation, or a dull ache.

4. *Duration*: In acute osteomyelitis, the duration is very short, whereas in chronic osteomyelitis, the disease may go on and on for many months or even years.

5. *Sinuses*: These may be present in chronic osteomyelitis either pyogenic or tuberculous. History of extrusion of bone chips is strongly suggestive of pyogenic osteomyelitis.

6. *Similar swellings*: Similar swellings elsewhere in the body usually indicate a case of diaphyseal aclasis, when multiple swellings may be seen arising from the metaphyses of different bones in a young boy.

K M. Iyer, *Clinical Examination in Orthopedics*,
DOI 10.1007/978-0-85729-971-0_1, © Springer-Verlag London Limited 2012

7. *Past history*: This is usually seen in otitis media, pneumonia, or typhoid fever in cases of acute osteomyelitis.
8. *Family history*: This may be useful and positive in certain bone diseases such as osteogenesis imperfecta congenita, achondroplasia, diaphyseal aclasis, etc.

General Survey

This may be helpful in certain cases when (1) anemia, with malnutrition may be seen in cases of secondary carcinomas and (2) toxic features of fever with malaise may be seen in acute osteomyelitis. The general survey may be completed in the following stages:

1. *Local examination*:

    (a) *Swelling*: The exact location and dimensions of the swelling are noted. All swellings arising from bone will be fixed to bone.
    (b) *Skin ov*erlying the swelling: In acute osteomyelitis, the overlying skin may be inflamed, tense, and shiny, whereas in tuberculous osteomyelitis, an initial cold abscess may be seen with sinus formation later on. Chronic osteomyelitis is usually seen with multiple sinuses. The tuberculous sinus will show characteristic features of an undermined edge along with a bluish tinge, whereas in chronic osteomyelitis, the presence of sprouting granulation tissue may be indicative of a sequestrum in its depth. A depressed and puckered scar may be indicative of a previous suppuration with abscess formation.
    (c) *Pressure effects*: This is particularly observed distal to the swelling in the limbs. There may be pressure giving rise to edema due to pressure on the veins, or there may be paresis due to involvement of the nerves.
    (d) *Neighboring joints*: Sympathetic effusion is usually common in acute osteomyelitis, which in certain cases may destroy the epiphyseal cartilage thus interfering with the growth of the bone.
    (e) *Muscular wasting*: This is very prominent and usually only seen in tuberculous osteomyelitis.
    (f) *Limb length* discrepancy: In certain infections, this feature may be seen resulting in growth of the affected bone, or destruction of the epiphyseal cartilage may result in arrest of the growth of the bone.

2. *Palpation*:

    (a) Local temperature: This is best felt with the back of the fingers; it is raised in acute osteomyelitis.
    (b) *T*enderness: Inflammatory swellings are normally tender, while bone tumors are generally non-tender.
    (c) Swelling: All swellings are invariably fixed to the bone underneath and the following points should be noted:

(i) *Situation*: The exact location of the swelling, such as the epiphyses in an osteoclastoma, the metaphyses in acute osteomyelitis, or the diaphyses as seen in Ewing's tumor.
(ii) *Size and shape*: A swelling which is diffuse and very difficult to delineate at its margins due to extreme pain may be due to inflammatory conditions. Pedunculated swellings are usually seen in exostoses, whereas spherical ovoid and irregular swellings may be seen in bone tumors.
(iii) *Surface*: A smooth and lobulated surface is usually seen in benign growths, while an irregular surface may be seen in cases of malignant growths or chronic infection.
(iv) *Edge*: An ill-defined edge may be seen in inflammatory swellings, while a well-defined edge may be seen in a new growth.
(v) *Consistency*: The swelling is usually bony hard in an osteoma, and exhibits features of "egg shell cracking" in an osteoclastoma. In osteosarcoma, the consistency varies, and it may be bony hard in certain places and soft in other places. In acute osteomyelitis, it may pit on pressure.
(vi) *Pulsation*: Some pathological conditions may be pulsatile such as a hemangioma of the bone or highly vascular osteoclastomas.

(d) *Bony irregularity*: This feature may be present in the neighboring surrounding bone in chronic osteomyelitis, syphilitic osteomyelitis, and even in tuberculous osteomyelitis.
(e) *Ulcers and sinuses*: It can be noted by lifting the base of the ulcer whether it is fixed to bone or can be moved against the bone. These are commonly seen in chronic pyogenic osteomyelitis or tuberculous osteomyelitis.
(f) *Presence of fracture*: In some cases this may be the presenting feature, as seen in primary carcinoma of the lungs, kidneys, breast, prostate, etc.
(g) *Neighboring structures*: These are examined as a matter of routine, for in some cases the neighboring structures may also be involved by the lesion.

3. *Percussion*: In a Brodie's abscess, striking with a fist may elicit tenderness over the spine and pelvis.
4. *Auscultation*: This feature may be helpful in detecting a murmur in pulsatile swellings.
5. *Measurements*: Two important measurements must always accompany the clinical examination, namely (a) the length of the bone and (b) the circumference of the affected limb if muscular wasting is suspected.
6. *Examination of the neighboring joints*: This may be valuable in detecting sympathetic effusion in acute osteomyelitis.
7. Examination of the lymph nodes.
8. *Pressure effects*: This may be seen in different locations of the body, such as in a "foot drop" due to paralysis of the lateral popliteal nerve which is seen in tumors of the upper end of the fibula.

General Examination

1. In cases of tuberculous osteomyelitis, the case history will include cough, evening rise of temperature, pain in the chest or haemoptysis, etc.
2. In syphilitic osteomyelitis, a case history must be completed regarding syphilitic contact, as well as an examination for evidence of other syphilitic stigmas on the body.
3. In cases of osteomyelitis, a search must also be made for other infective foci in the skin, teeth, tonsils, ears, etc.
4. Certain bony lesions may also involve other bones: e.g., diaphyseal aclasis, etc.
5. In cases of secondary carcinoma, a complete, thorough examination must be made of thyroid, kidneys, lungs, prostate, breast, uterus, etc.

Special Investigations

1. *Blood*: A full blood count to include hemoglobin %, white blood cell count total and differential, erythrocyte sedimentation rate, and plasma proteins, along with serum electrolytes and serum calcium and phosphorus estimates, is done in every case. Serum acid and alkaline phosphatase along with Wassermann reaction and Kahn tests are also done to be extremely sure.
2. *Urine*: Estimation of albumin and protein, along with the A/G ratio and the presence of Bence Jones protein, are also noted.
3. *X-ray examination*: This is initially done of the affected bone and later extended to other bones in certain cases when generalized diseases are suspected. The initial plain radiographs are done in anteroposterior and lateral directions to identify the lesion with greater accuracy (Fig. 1.1). Certain X-rays show characteristic changes such as in diaphyseal aclasis, multiple exostoses are seen. An expansile lesion situated in the metaphyseal-epiphyseal region with its cavity traversed by bony trabeculae giving a soap-bubble appearance is characteristic of an osteoclastoma (Fig. 1.2). An osteosarcoma may show a characteristic sunburst appearance with sun-ray spicules and a wedge-shaped area of ossification called the Codman's triangle where the periosteum is elevated. X-ray examination of other bones is usually done when rickets, Paget's disease or multiple myeloma is suspected. In all cases, the lungs are X-rayed as a routine part of the examination.
4. *Arteriography*: This may be useful in certain cases when the blood vessels supplying a tumor are tortuous and engorged.
5. *Radioactive scanning*: Technetium-99m polyphosphate scanning is usually preferred because of its ability to detect early active lesions in bone before they are visible on X-rays.
6. *Biopsy*: This is mandatory in suspicious lesions. Biopsies are of various types. An open biopsy is the preferred choice rather than an aspiration or marrow biopsy.

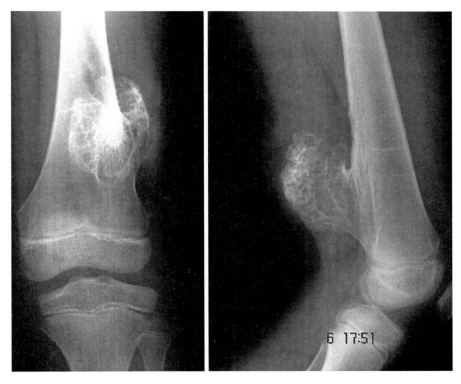

Fig. 1.1 Anteroposterior and lateral radiographs showing an osteochondroma (exostosis) of the lower end of the femur (Courtesy Dilip Malhotra, Bahrain)

7. *Bacteriological examination*: This is extremely useful when pus is obtained, to determine the exact nature of the organism. In certain cases, blood culture may be useful in suspected cases of septicemia.
8. Histopathological examination of the tumor material obtained by biopsy or marrow biopsy is very useful in certain cases.

Classification of Bony Swellings

1. *Traumatic*: These may be seen in excess callus formation from a fractured bone, a malunited fracture or myositis ossificans, or a subperiosteal hematoma and its ossification.
2. *Inflammatory*: As seen in acute osteomyelitis, chronic osteomyelitis, Brodie's abscess, typhoid osteomyelitis, tuberculous osteomyelitis, syphilitic osteitis, and pneumococcal osteomyelitis.

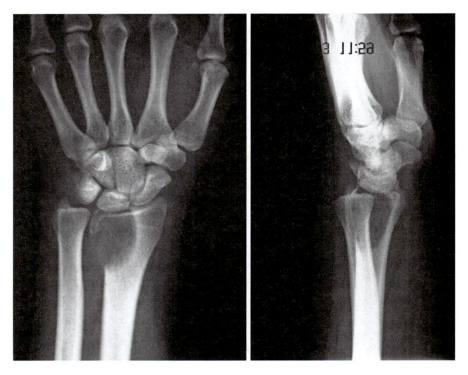

Fig. 1.2 Anteroposterior and lateral radiographs of the wrist showing a giant cell tumour of the distal radius (Courtesy Dilip Malhotra, Bahrain)

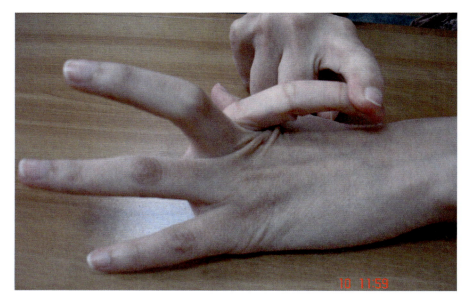

Fig. 1.3 Clinical photograph showing hyperlaxity of ligaments as in Marfan's syndrome (Courtesy Dilip Malhotra, Bahrain)

Fig. 1.4 Anteroposterior radiograph of the knee showing an unicameral bone cyst of the proximal fibula (Courtesy Dilip Malhotra, Bahrain)

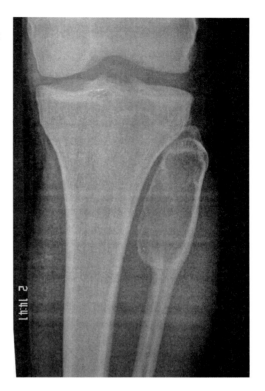

3. *Developmental disorders*: These may be seen in achondroplasia, osteogenesis imperfecta, mucopolysaccharide disorders, Morquio-Brailsford disease, Hurler's disease, diaphyseal aclasis, multiple enchondromas, marble bones, candle bones, spotted bones, striped bones, cleidocranial dysostosis, and fibrous dysplasia.

4. Nutritional, metabolic, and endocrine disorders as seen in rickets, osteomalacia, scurvy, hyperparathyroidism, and osteoporosis.

5. *Malformation syndromes*: These include nail-patella syndrome, Marfan's syndrome (Fig. 1.3), and Paget's disease.

6. *Cyst*: This is seen in a solitary cyst (Fig. 1.4), cyst associated with generalized osteitis fibrosa, hydatid cyst, and an aneurysmal bone cyst.

7. *Tumors*:

   (a) Benign tumors such as osteoma, osteochondroma, osteoblastoma, osteoid osteoma, chondroma, chondroblastoma, periosteal fibroma, fibroma, chondromyxoid fibroma, hemangioma, lipoma and neurofibroma.

   (b) *Locally malignant tumor*: osteoclastoma (giant cell tumor; Fig. 1.2).

   (c) *Malignant tumors*:

- *Primary*: osteosarcoma, chondrosarcoma, Ewing's tumor, multiple myeloma, reticulum cell sarcoma, plasmacytoma, fibrosarcoma, liposarcoma, and angiosarcoma.
- *Secondary*: carcinoma of bone by primary carcinoma metastasis from thyroid, bronchus, breast, prostate, kidney, uterus, gastrointestinal tract, testis, or other, or by direct infiltration from adjacent growths – e.g., carcinoma of the tongue involving the lower jaw.

Chapter 2
Examination of the Shoulder

The shoulder girdle consists of three joints and one articulation – namely:

1. The sternoclavicular joint
2. The acromioclavicular joint
3. The glenohumeral or shoulder joint and
4. The scapulothoracic articulation.

Inspection

Asymmetry of the shoulder is very obvious when examined by bilateral compression of the two shoulder joints. This may be very easily noticed when the arm is hanging down the side, if it is internally rotated and adducted, as in Erb's palsy, like a waiter receiving a tip.

The deltoid region is next inspected as it is normally full and round, but may be vacant as in cases of anterior shoulder dislocation. The arm is then held slightly away from the trunk (Fig. 2.1).

The deltopectoral groove is located just medial to the shoulder mass, between the anterior fibers of the deltoid and the pectoralis major, and it contains the cephalic vein which can be used for a venous cutdown. It is also a very important site for incisions in the shoulder region.

Over the posterior aspect of the shoulder girdle is the most prominent part which is the scapula. This is very easy to locate as it is situated over the ribs two to seven in the resting position, and its medial border is nearly 2 in. away from the spinous processes. Occasionally the scapula has only partially descended from the neck to the thorax resulting in a Sprengel's deformity. Occasionally the midline spinous processes may show a lateral scoliotic deformity resulting in elevation or depression of the shoulders. Very rarely do the spinous processes show a rounded kyphotic deformity due to Scheuermann's disease in adolescents.

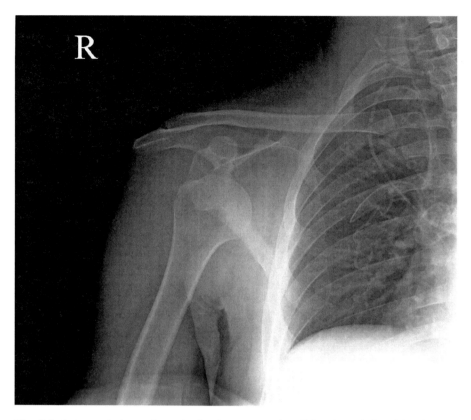

Fig. 2.1 Anteroposterior radiograph showing an anterior dislocation of the right shoulder (Courtesy Dilip Malhotra, Bahrain)

Palpation

Bony landmarks can be palpated systematically by beginning from the suprasternal notch. The joint that is immediately lateral is the sternoclavicular joint which is best appreciated when palpated bilaterally. The clavicle is normally slightly superior to the manubrium sternum, and it rises from it. Dislocations of the sternoclavicular joint are frequently seen when the clavicle has shifted over the manubrium sternum. Proceeding with the palpation laterally, the clavicle represents a medial convex smooth surface which is well felt in its full length, becoming concave at its lateral end. The lateral end of the clavicle forms the coracoid process which faces anterolaterally and lies deep under cover of the pectoralis major muscle. The acromioclavicular joint lies immediately lateral to the coracoid process and can be easily felt by asking the patient to flex and extend his or her shoulder several times. This joint may be prominent and tender in dislocations of the lateral end of the clavicle. Palpating just lateral to the acromioclavicular joint, one finds the acromion process. Continuing palpation just lateral to the acromion and slightly inferiorly, one reaches the greater tuberosity of the humerus. The bicipital grove is located just medial and anterior to the greater tuberosity and is best felt when the arm is externally rotated, when the tendon of the long head of the biceps can be rolled. Palpating posteriorly and medially, one finds the acromion tapering into the spine of the scapula as one continuous arch. The medial border of the scapula is about 2 in. from the spinous process of the thoracic vertebrae, and the triangle at the medial end of the spine of the scapula is at L3 level.

The soft tissue palpation is mainly into four regions, namely (1) the rotator cuff, (2) the subacromial and subdeltoid bursa, (3) the axilla, and (4) the muscles around the shoulder girdle.

1. *The rotator cuff*: This cuff is composed mainly of three muscles which form an insertion into the greater tuberosity of the humerus – namely, the supraspinatus, the infraspinatus, and the teres minor. The fourth muscle is the subscapularis which is located anteriorly. The rotator cuff is clinically important because the supraspinatus is the most commonly ruptured muscle near its insertion.
2. The subacromial bursa has two main components – namely, the subacromial and the subdeltoid parts. This is a frequent pathologic finding causing tenderness and limitation of shoulder movements.
3. The axilla is a pyramidal space through which nerves and vessels pass into the upper arm. Enlarged lymph nodes can be well palpated in this space. The axilla is formed anteriorly by the pectoralis major muscle and posteriorly by the latissimus dorsi muscle, while its medial wall is formed by the second to sixth ribs with its overlying serratus anterior muscle, and the lateral wall is limited by the bicipital groove of the humerus. The shoulder joint is the apex of the pyramid, and the axilla is supplied by the brachial plexus and the axillary arteries.
4. The muscles of the shoulder girdle:
   The sternocleidomastoid is palpated on the side opposite to which the head is turned and is mainly important for hematomas in the muscle which can cause a wry neck, swollen lymph nodes due to infection, and may frequently be traumatized in injuries of the neck, such as a whiplash injury.
   The pectoralis major muscle is very important clinically as it may be absent congenitally, most frequently either in whole or in part. The costochondral junctions which lie just next to the sternum are the frequent site of costochondritis when they are tender on palpation.
   The biceps muscle is palpated with the elbow in resisted flexion and can be seen curled up in the midarm when the long head of the biceps is torn. The long head of the biceps may be involved in tenosynovitis when it is tender or may be dislocated in the bicipital grove which is well palpated when the shoulder is laterally rotated.

The deltoid may be atrophied in cases of axillary nerve damage usually because of shoulder dislocations. The deltoid muscle converges down to the midpoint of the lateral aspect of the arm to a bony prominence known as the deltoid tuberosity.

The trapezius is a fan-shaped muscle which extends from the occiput along the spinous processes of the cervical spine into the clavicle, acromion, and the spine of the scapula where it merges into the origin of the deltoid.

The rhomboids retract the scapulae and run from the spinous processes of the cervical spine vertebrae obliquely downward and laterally, to insert into the medial border of the scapula. They can be palpated by asking the patient to put his arm behind his back with the elbows flexed and the arms internally rotated when the patient pushes posteriorly as this movement is resisted.

The latissimus dorsi has a broad origin at the iliac crest and twists upon itself toward the shoulder before being inserted into the floor of the bicipital groove of the humerus.

The serratus anterior muscle prevents winging of the scapula by anchoring the medial border of the scapula to the thoracic cage.

Range of Movements

The range of movements possible in the shoulder girdle are mainly abduction, adduction, flexion, extension, internal rotation, and lateral rotation. These movements are tested both actively and passively.

The Apley's scratch test evaluates all the ranges of movements of the shoulder girdle. Firstly, ask the patient to touch the superomedial angle of the opposite scapula behind her head. This tests abduction and lateral rotation. Next ask the patient to touch the opposite acromion in front of her head, which tests internal rotation and adduction. Finally, further test adduction and internal rotation by asking the patient to touch the opposite scapula at its inferior angle, from behind.

Another way in which all of these movements are tested is by asking the patient to abduct his arm to 90° while keeping the elbows extended. Then, with his forearms supinated, ask him to carry on abduction at the shoulders until the palms touch each other over the top of the head, which tests full bilateral abduction at the shoulders. Next ask the patient to keep his hands behind his neck and push his elbows posteriorly which tests abduction and lateral rotations. Finally, ask the patient to keep his hands behind his back as high as they will go to test for adduction and internal rotations.

The glenohumeral joint is tested passively through its full range, but when it has a full passive range but is limited in its active range, that signifies that muscular weakness is the problem.

To differentiate between extra and intra-articular block, feeling at the point of blockage will determine which is involved: It is rubbery in cases of soft tissue extra-articular block, as compared with a bony block which is abrupt and bony in nature.

All of these active and passive movements are tested in three different stages: namely, pure glenohumeral motion, scapulothoracic motion, and a combination of both.

1. *Abduction/adduction*: This occurs in a ratio of 2:1 at the glenohumeral joint and the scapulothoracic joint. It is normally 180° and 45° at both the joints. Another way to test this is by firmly anchoring the scapula and then testing for abduction, when the pure glenohumeral movement is about 90° at which point the scapula begins to move, which can be felt. Full abduction is completed when the arm is externally rotated so as to increase the articulating surface of the humeral head.

In cases of a frozen shoulder, the movement occurs mainly by scapulothoracic movement and never in the glenohumeral joint.

2. *Flexion/extension*: Normal movement is about 90° for flexion and 45° for extension. These movements may be limited in cases of bursitis of the shoulder or bicipital tendinitis.
3. *Internal rotation/external rotation*: This is best tested by keeping the elbows close to the waist which prevents substitutions of rotation, and flexing the elbows to 90° and then rotating the arm laterally and medially. The normal range of internal rotation is about 55°, and the normal range of external rotation is about 45°. The alternative technique to test for internal and external rotations is by asking the patient to abduct both her shoulders to 90° with bent elbows to 90° and then test for rotations with palms facing upward and downward.

Neurologic Examination

This is mainly done through tests in the shoulder girdle: namely, flexion, extension, abduction, adduction, external rotation, internal rotation, scapular elevation, scapular retraction, and shoulder protraction.

1. *Flexors*:
   (a) Primary flexors – anterior fibers of the deltoid
       – Axillary nerve – C5
       – Coracobrachialis-musculocutaneous nerve – C5, C6.
   (b) Secondary flexors – pectoralis major (clavicular head)
       – Biceps
       – Anterior fibers of deltoid.
   Flexion is tested by flexing the elbow to 90° and then starting flexion of the shoulder. Gradually and slowly increase resistance as flexion at the shoulder begins (Table 2.1).
2. *Extensors*:
   (a) Primary extensors – latissimus dorsi – thoracodorsal nerve – C6, C7, C8
       – Teres major-lower scapular nerve – C5, C6
       – Posterior fibers of the deltoid – axillary nerve – C5, C6

Table 2.1 Muscle grading chart

Muscle gradations	Description
5 Normal	Complete range of motion against gravity with full resistance
4 Good	Complete range of motion against gravity with some resistance
3 Fair	Complete range of motion against gravity
2 Poor	Complete range of motion with gravity eliminated
1 Trace	Evidence of slight contractility. No joint motion
0 Zero	No evidence of contractility

(b) Secondary extensors – teres minor
  – Triceps (long head)

Test for extension by gradually increasing resistance to flexion over the posterior aspect of the distal humerus (Table 2.1).

3. *Abduction*:
  (a) Primary abductors – middle fibers of the deltoid – axillary nerve – C5, C6
    – Supraspinatus-suprascapular nerve – C5, C6
  (b) Secondary abductors – anterior and posterior fibers of the deltoid
    – Serratus anterior

This is tested by asking the patient to abduct his arm against gradually increasing resistance.

4. *Adduction*:
  (a) Primary adductors – pectoralis major-medial and lateral anterior thoracic nerve – C5, C6, C7, C8, T1
    – Latissimus dorsi-thoracodorsal nerve – C6, C7, C8
  (b) Secondary adductors – teres major
    – Anterior fibers of the deltoid

This is tested by adduction of a slightly abducted arm against gradually increasing resistance offered on the medial side of the arm.

5. *External rotation*:
  (a) Primary external rotators
    – Infraspinatus-suprascapular nerve – C5, C6
    – Teres minor – branch of the axillary nerve – C5
  (b) Secondary external rotators
    – Posterior fibers of the deltoid

This is tested by holding a flexed elbow at the waist with the forearm in a neutral position and asking the patient to rotate her arm outward against gradually increasing resistance.

6. *Internal rotators*:
  (a) Primary internal rotators
    – Subscapularis – upper and lower subscapular nerves – C5, C6
    – Pectoralis major – medial and lateral anterior thoracic nerves – C5, C6, C7, C8, T1
    – Latissimus dorsi – thoracodorsal nerve – C6, C7, C8
    – Teres major – lower subscapular nerve – C5, C6
  (b) Secondary internal rotator
    – Posterior fibers of the deltoid

The test is carried out in the same way as above, and the patient is asked to rotate his arm inward against gradually increasing resistance.

7. *Scapular elevation*:
  (a) Primary elevators
    – The trapezius-spinal accessory nerve or cranial nerve XI
    – Levator scapulae – C3, C4 along with branches from the dorsal scapular nerve, C5
  (b) Secondary elevators
    – Rhomboid major
    – Rhomboid minor

Ask the patient to shrug his shoulders against gradually increasing resistance.

8. *Scapular retraction*:
   (a) Primary retractors – rhomboid major – dorsal scapular nerve – C5
       – Rhomboid minor – dorsal scapular nerve – C5
   (b) Secondary retractors – the trapezius
   This can be tested by asking the patient to throw his shoulders back against gradually increasing resistance, whereby the patient assumes a position of attention.
9. *Scapular protraction*:
   (a) The primary protractor is the serratus anterior – long thoracic nerve – C5, C6, C7
   This is tested by asking the patient to reach forward when the scapula moves anteriorly on the thorax. Winging is seen when the patient pushes against a wall or when doing a push-up, when the serratus anterior is weak.

Reflex Testing

Both the muscles, biceps, and triceps which cross the shoulder joint should be tested.

Sensation Testing

These can be tested by well-delineated dermatomes as follows:

1. The lateral arm – C5 nerve root – which is examined by a rounded area just on the lateral aspect of the deltoid muscle – axillary nerve.
2. The medial arm, supplied by the T1 nerve root.
3. The axilla which is supplied by the T2 nerve root.
4. The area from the axilla to the nipple is supplied by the T3 nerve root.
5. The nipple which is supplied by the T4 nerve root.

Abnormal sensations (paresthesia) may either be increased (hyperesthesia) or decreased (hypoesthesia) or may be completely absent (anesthesia). The axillary nerve is frequently damaged in shoulder dislocations, when it leaves an anesthetic patch over the lateral aspect of the deltoid muscle.

Special Tests

Certain special tests are helpful in the examination of the shoulder girdle.

1. The Yergason test which is performed to test for the stability of the long head of the biceps. This is done by externally rotating the arm as the patient resists and at the same time pulling downward on his elbow. If the biceps tendon is unstable, it will jump out of the groove giving rise to pain.
2. *Drop arm test*: This is done by asking the patient to abduct her arm and then slowly lowering it arm to her side. This test is mainly for integrity of the rotators, and if those are damaged or torn, the arm drops off after abduction to fall by the side.

3. *Apprehension test*: This is mainly an indication of anxiety while testing for the integrity in a movement toward dislocating a shoulder, which is seen on the patient's facial expression while doing the test. This test is done by abduction and external rotation of the arm in an attempt to dislocate the shoulder.

Examination of Related Areas

The shoulder joint area is the site for referred pain in certain conditions, which must be borne in mind.

Shoulder symptoms due to an irritated diaphragm being supplied by the same nerve root innervations (C4, C5) may be seen in a myocardial infarction. Certain problems such as a prolapsed cervical disc may be referred to the medial angle of the scapula. Occasionally a spinal fracture may have radiation to the shoulder along its muscle inserted into the scapula. Sometimes pain may radiate retrograde proximally in cases of injuries to the distal humerus or the elbow.

Certain specific conditions affecting the shoulder joint should be borne in mind, such as:

1. Scapular disorders such as:

   (a) *Sprengel's shoulder*: Sometimes one scapula remains high due to incomplete descent from the neck, which is usually around the third month of fetal life. In these cases, deformity along with limitation of movements is the only symptom, along with a web of skin which runs along the side of the neck. Radiographs may show an extra bony mass (omovertebral) between the upper scapula and the cervical spine. Mild cases are left untreated, and excision of the superomedial part of the scapula may help in reducing the deformity.

   (b) *Winged scapula*: This is a condition seen in paralysis of the serratus anterior. Winging along with backward projection of the vertebral border of the scapula becomes obvious when the patient is asked to push his hands against the wall. The disability is very slight and is best accepted without treatment.

   (c) *Grating scapula*: This is a painless and noisy or grating sound which is heard when arm movements are attempted, and no treatment is advised for this condition.

2. Tuberculosis of the shoulder:
   This is usually seen in advanced cases, and when there is no discharge, the term 'caries sicca" is used. This condition usually mimics a frozen shoulder in many cases, with overall decrease of all movements, with pain. On radiography, generalized rarefaction is seen. Treatment is generally by resting the shoulder in an abduction splint, resulting in decrease of pain and healing by fibrosis. Very rarely a clearance operation is indicated, if the symptoms do not settle.

3. *Musculotendinous cuff lesions*:
   The rotator cuff comprising the supraspinatus, infraspinatus, subscapularis, and the teres minor may show varying pathology in its tendinous portions, such as degeneration, trauma with tears, and a reaction of inflammation indicative of repair.

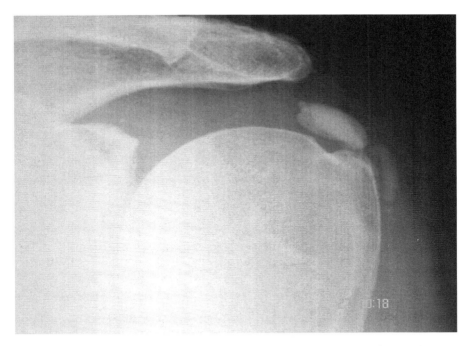

Fig. 2.2 Anteroposterior radiograph of the shoulder showing supraspinatus calcification (Courtesy Dilip Malhotra, Bahrain)

In acute tendinitis, degeneration is usually seen as a small localized area in the supraspinatus tendon due to deposition of calcium. This is usually seen in younger adults with a markedly painful shoulder along with marked decrease in range of movement. Radiographs may show a dense area of calcification just above the greater tuberosity (Fig. 2.2). Treatment is by rest in a sling, along with analgesics. Very rarely is aspiration of the calcific mass necessary under image-intensifier control.

In chronic tendinitis or the painful arc syndrome, the patient is usually older, and only certain movements of the shoulder are painful, such as in the mid arc of abduction. This is usually treated by conservative measures such as rest, along with heat. In refractory cases, an injection of hydrocortisone along with a local anesthetic is helpful. Very rarely is operative treatment in the form of an acromionectomy indicated.

4. *Frozen shoulder*:

This is a fairly common condition, which is also known as adhesive capsulitis or periarthritis of the shoulder. It usually starts in the supraspinatus tendon and gradually spreads to involve the entire tendinous cuff. Initially there is pain, which gradually settles down, along with limitation of all movements, both active and passive. This condition must be differentiated from posttraumatic stiffness, tuberculosis, and osteoarthritis. Treatment of this condition is usually conservative in the form of rest, analgesics, and heat in the form of short-wave diathermy. Exercises are gradually encouraged and at times an injection of hydrocortisone along with a local anesthetic may be helpful. In extremely refractory cases, a manipulation under an anesthetic may hasten recovery.

5. *Supraspinatus tears*:
   This may be partial or complete, and it usually follows degeneration in the tendon. The patient may gradually recover if it is a partial tear, when the pain subsides. When complete, the pain subsides, but active abduction is impossible, and the patient demonstrates a characteristic shrug, whereas passive abduction is possible above a right angle, but cannot be held, thus allowing the shoulder to drop. Treatment of this condition depends on whether the tear is partial or complete. Partial tears are usually treated by rest, analgesics, exercises, and injections of hydrocortisone with a local anesthetic. When the tear is complete, surgical repair is always desirable.

6. *Lesions of the biceps tendon*:

   (a) *Tendinitis*: This is fairly common, with the shoulder joint normal with tenderness which is felt in the bicipital groove only on external rotation. This condition usually responds to rest, local heat, and injections of hydrocortisone along with a local anesthetic.
   (b) *Ruptured biceps tendon*: This is due to a tear of the long head of the biceps, with the tendon usually being avulsed from its insertion. The clinical picture is characteristic: On asking the patient to flex both his elbows, the belly of the biceps is lower and more rounded when compared with the opposite normal side. Usually this is often left alone, but occasionally it may be repaired in patients engaged in heavy manual labor.

7. *Brachial neuralgia*:
   This is a term which is usually applied to pain extending over a large part of the upper limb. It can be conveniently classified on an anatomical basis into three parts:

   (a) Disorders around the shoulder: In all of these conditions, the shoulder joint movements are limited and painful.
   (b) Disorders proximal to the shoulder: In all of these cases, the shoulder joint movements are essentially normal along with a normal radiographic appearance.
   (c) Disorders distal to the shoulder: In all of these cases, the shoulder joint and the neck movements are normal along with a normal radiographic appearance. Lesions such as tennis elbow and carpal tunnel syndrome must be kept in mind.

Chapter 3
Examination of the Elbow

The elbow is a hinge joint comprising three main articulations – namely:

1. The humeroulnar joint
2. The humeroradial joint and
3. The radioulnar joint.

Inspection

Inspection of the elbow joint is by means of observing the carrying angle, swelling, and scars. When the elbow joint is extended in the normal anatomic position with the palms facing anteriorly, the longitudinal axis of the forearm is at a slight valgus (lateral) deviation to the longitudinal axis of the arm. This is known as the carrying angle of the elbow, which is normally 5° in males and between 10° and 15° in females, as it allows for the elbow to fit into the depression at the waist immediately above the iliac crest. Cubitus valgus occurs when this carrying angle is increased to more than normal, as in epiphyseal injuries of the lateral condyle, which usually presents as a delayed ulnar nerve palsy due to gradual stretching of the ulnar nerve. Cubitus varus is seen when the carrying angle is less than normal with deviation of the forearm medially behind the body. It is also called the "gunstock" deformity which is commonly caused by a malunited supracondylar fracture of the distal humerus in a child. This deformity is more frequently seen than the cubitus valgus deformity.

Swellings around the elbow joint may be localized or diffuse in nature. It may be localized, as in cases of olecranon bursitis where it is limited by the bursa. Trauma to the elbow may result in a diffuse swelling around the elbow joint and arm and upper forearm. In both these cases, the creases of the elbow are lost. Scars may seen in the anterior aspect of the elbow joint over the cubital region due to repeated needle pricks, including by drug addicts.

K M. Iyer, *Clinical Examination in Orthopedics*,
DOI 10.1007/978-0-85729-971-0_3, © Springer-Verlag London Limited 2012

Palpation

Palpation is carried out by bony palpation followed by soft tissue palpation. Crepitus is localized by bony palpation and is seen in osteoarthritis and fractures which may be synovial or bursal in origin. The bony landmarks are palpated in a sequential manner as follows: The medial epicondyle is easily palpable at the medial side of the distal end of the humerus as it is subcutaneous throughout and is commonly tender in fractures in children. Palpating moving upwards, one finds a small bony ridge which is covered by the thick origin of the wrist flexor muscles. Very rarely a small bony process may be felt which is compressing the median nerve causing symptoms of median nerve compression. The olecranon is a large process at the superior end of the ulna, and along its length it is subcutaneous in nature. At its superior end, its bursa is situated. The ulnar border of the ulna can be palpated throughout its entire length until the level of the ulnar styloid process at the wrist joint. The olecranon fossa lies at the distal end of the posterior aspect of the humerus, which accommodates the olecranon during extension of the elbow joint. It is normally filled with fat and is best palpated with the elbow in partial extension. The lateral epicondyle is located just lateral to the olecranon and is smaller and less well defined than the medial epicondyle. Palpating upwards, one finds the lateral supracondylar ridge until the deltoid tubercle, which is more well defined and longer than the medial supracondylar ridge. With the elbow flexed to 90°, the medial epicondyle, the tip of the olecranon and the lateral epicondyle form an isosceles triangle. These form a straight line when the elbow is extended. With the patient's arm abducted and the elbow held flexed in 90°, if he can perform supination and pronation, more than three quarters of the radial head can be palpable. This may be seen easily in radial head dislocations.

Soft tissue palpation can be divided into four zones: namely, the medial area, the posterior aspect, the lateral aspect, and the anterior aspect.

In the medial zone, the most important structure to be palpated is the ulnar nerve, which is located in the sulcus behind the medial epicondyle and the olecranon. This, when rolled between the fingers, is round, soft, and tubular in nature. This nerve when rolled against the ulnar groove elicits a "funny bone" sensation. It may be thickened in early indications of leprosy. The nerve may be injured in a supracondylar fracture or in cases of direct trauma.

Wrist flexor-pronator muscle group: This group mainly consists of four muscles: namely, the pronator teres, flexor carpi radialis, palmaris longus, and flexor carpi ulnaris, all of which originate as a common conjoined tendon from the medial epicondyle. This origin may be strained in activities requiring pronation, such as tennis and golf or using a screwdriver. The pronator teres is not separately palpable as it is deep and covered by other muscles. The flexor carpi radialis is tested by asking the patient to make a fist and radially deviate the wrist first, followed by palmar flexion of the wrist, when it is palpated just radial to the palmaris longus at the wrist. The palmar longus is tested as described in Chap. 4 on examination of the hand and wrist. Finally, the flexor carpi ulnaris can be tested by the patient making a fist: the muscle stands out on the ulnar side of the palmaris longus just proximal to the pisiform.

The medial collateral ligament extends from the epicondyle until the medial margin of the ulnar notch of the trochlea.

Supracondylar nodes are very clearly felt along the medial supracondylar line. If they are slippery to the touch, that mainly indicates an infection in the hand or forearm.

Over the posterior aspect of the soft tissue of the elbow is palpated the triceps muscle and the olecranon bursa. The triceps muscle, as its name implies, originates from three heads, namely, the long, lateral and the medial heads. The long head crosses the glenohumeral and the elbow joints, and together with the lateral and medial heads, it forms an aponeurosis which is broad and fans out to be inserted into the olecranon. The olecranon bursa overlies the olecranon and may be inflamed giving rise to a classic bursitis, which is aptly called student's elbow.

The next zone is the lateral aspect of the elbow: This has a common origin from the lateral humeral epicondyle and consists of the brachioradialis, the extensor carpi radialis longus and the extensor carpi radialis brevis. The brachioradialis muscle is tested by asking the patient to make a fist while placing it on the table and raising it against resistance, when it is palpated at its insertion just close to the radial styloid process. The extensor carpi radialis longus and brevis are palpated during wrist extension when they is delineated just proximal to the second and third metacarpals. This common extensor origin is commonly strained in "tennis elbow" when there is pain centered over the lateral epicondyle and also along the course of these muscles when tested by resisted extension of the wrist. The lateral collateral ligament is a rope-like structure which extends from the lateral epicondyle to the side of the annular ligament of the head of the radius. The annular ligament is attached to the lateral ligament, and it encircles the head and neck of the radius holding it and permitting it to articulate with the ulna.

The anterior zone forms the cubital fossa which is a triangular space with the brachioradialis on its lateral border and the pronator teres on its medial border. The base of this triangular space is formed by a straight line joining the two epicondyles of the humerus. It contains the following four structures from the lateral to the medial borders: The biceps tendon can be palpated by asking the patient to place a closed fist supinated on the examining table, when it is felt as like a taut chord just medial to the brachioradialis. A ruptured biceps tendon is a commonly seen condition, and presents with a tender cubital fossa with the muscle belly forming a bulbous swelling which retracts upwards in the upper arm as the muscle contracts. The sensation that can be felt just medial to the biceps tendon is the pulsation of the brachial artery. The median nerve lies just medial to the brachial artery. The musculocutaneous nerve lies just lateral to the biceps and supplies sensation to the forearm.

Range of Motion

Active range of movements: This is evaluated by the patient moving the elbow without assistance. Flexion is possible up to 135° when the patient tries to bend his hand, and extension is usually possible to 0°. It cannot be done beyond this because of biceps muscle tension.

Supination and pronation are tested by the patient holding a pencil, which is used as a marker in the fist of the arm with the flexed elbow. The patient is then asked to carry out pronation and supination, which are normally possible to 90° in either direction. These movements may be decreased in radioulnar synostosis or certain affections of the wrist and the elbow.

Passive range of movements: These are tested only when the patient is unable to perform the active tests. All of these must always be tested with the elbows beside the patient's body at the waist.

Neurologic Examination

This is done in three stages:
1. *Muscle testing*:
   (a) *Flexion*:
      (i)   Primary flexors – brachialis – musculocutaneous nerve – C5, C6
         – Biceps when the forearm is supinated
         – Musculocutaneous nerve – C5, C6
      (ii) Secondary flexors – brachioradialis
         – Supinator

This is tested by asking the patient to flex the arm slowly while increasing resistance.
   (b) *Extension*:
      (i)   Primary extensor – triceps – radial nerve – C7
      (ii) Secondary extensor – anconeus

This is tested by asking the patient to gently extend his elbow against resistance.
   (c) *Supination*:
      (i)   *Primary supinators*:
         – Biceps – musculocutaneous nerve – C5, C6
         – Supinator-radial nerve – C6
      (ii) *Secondary supinator*:
         – Brachioradialis
   (d) *Pronation*:
      (i)   *Primary pronators*:
         – Pronator teres – median nerve – C6
         – Pronator quadratus – anterior branch of the median nerve – C8, T1
      (ii) Secondary pronator – flexor carpi radialis

Both these movements are tested by asking the patient to pronate her forearm from the position of supination, gradually increasing resistance and vice versa.

2. *Reflex testing*:
There are three basic deep tendon reflexes, each being a lower motor neuron reflex that tests the innervations of the elbow joint.

The biceps reflex – C5 is tested by holding the forearm over the opposite arm such that it rests on your forearm. With the hand supporting the patient's arm on the medial side, place the thumb over the biceps tendon in the cubital fossa to elicit the jerk by tapping it. The biceps jerk is felt slightly in normal patients. An increased jerk is felt and seen in an upper motor neuron lesion such as a stroke, while a decreased response is seen and felt in a lower motor neuron lesion such as a peripheral nerve lesion in a prolapsed cervical disc.

The brachioradialis reflex – C6 is tested by tapping the distal end of the tendon at the radial styloid which elicits the reflex.

The triceps reflex – C7 is tested by tapping over the tendon of the triceps just as it crosses the olecranon fossa with the arm held relaxed in the bent position when the jerk is elicited.

3. *Sensation testing*:

(a) C5 *supplies the la*teral aspect of the arm through the sensory branches of the axillary nerve.
(b) C6 supplies the lateral aspect of the forearm through sensory branches of the musculocutaneous nerve.
(c) C8 supplies sensory branches to the medial forearm through the antebrachial cutaneous nerve.
(d) T1 supplies sensation to the medial arm through the brachial cutaneous nerve.

Special Tests

Special tests are done to test for ligamentous stability by holding the elbow in an extended position when a valgus or a varus strain can be given to provide for slight opening of the elbow joint on the opposite side.

Tinel sign is done to test the presence of a neuroma within a nerve like the ulnar nerve. Tapping the ulnar nerve between the olecranon and the neuroma in the groove will elicit a tingling sensation down the forearm to the hand.

The tennis elbow test is done reproduce sudden pain over the common extensor origin over the lateral epicondyle by resistance offered to the dorsum of the wrist in an attempt to flex the wrist into flexion. Sharp pain is experienced at the lateral epicondyle.

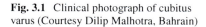

Fig. 3.1 Clinical photograph of cubitus varus (Courtesy Dilip Malhotra, Bahrain)

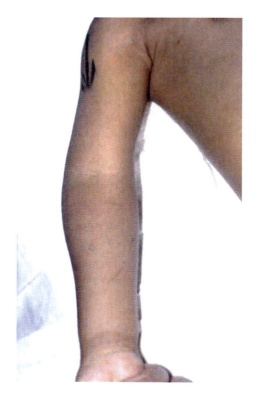

Examination of Related Areas

Cervical spine pathology and certain wrist affections may give referred pain at the elbow, as the wrist flexors and extensors cross both the elbow and wrist joints. Certain commonly seen conditions of the elbow must always be kept in mind.

1. *Elbow deformities*:

   (a) *Cubitus varus or gunstock deformity*: this deformity is fairly common and seen in a malunited supracondylar fracture. This is usually correctible by a wedge osteotomy of the lower distal humerus (Fig. 3.1).
   (b) *Cubitus valgus*: This is commonly seen in a malunited fracture of the lateral condyle. The deformity per se does not require any treatment but may require an anterior transposition of the ulnar nerve for delayed ulnar nerve palsy in some cases.
   (c) *Dislocated head of the radius*: This condition may be congenital or due to failure to reduce a pronation injury of the elbow. This condition may also be seen in certain bone dysplasias, when it is usually lateral. If the bony lump restricts elbow flexion, then the best treatment is to excise the radial head.

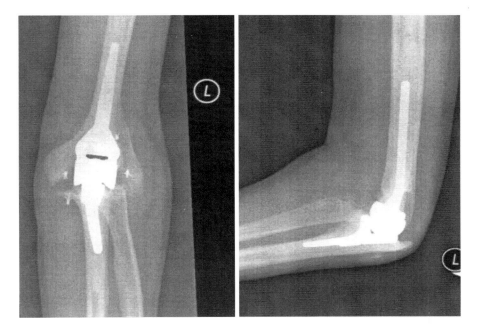

Fig. 3.2 Anteroposterior and lateral radiographs of the left elbow showing a total elbow replacement (Courtesy Dushyant H. Thakkar, London, UK)

2. *Stiffness of the elbows*:
   This may be seen in one or both elbows. When seen in both elbows, rheumatoid arthritis or other causes such as arthrogryposis multiplexa congenita and ankylosing spondylitis should be considered. It may become essential to treat one of the elbows by arthroplasty or joint replacement, to enable the hand to reach the mouth (Fig. 3.2). When seen in one elbow, congenital synostosis of the superior radioulnar joint must be kept in mind when there is also a loss of rotation.

   (a) *Posttraumatic stiffness*: This may be seen after any injury to the elbow. This is usually very severe, when seen with a lot of myositis ossificans. Removal of the myositis ossificans may be done in cases of bone block to flexion, but the gain in movements is not often very great.

   (b) *Tuberculosis*: Sinus formation is relatively common since the elbow is a superficial joint. The most striking physical sign is marked wasting in a swollen warm elbow that is held flexed. Radiographs also help in localizing the lesion. Treatment is toward the general condition along with rest and a removable polythene splint when healing occurs by fibrous tissue.

   (c) *Osteoarthritis*: This may result from damage to the articular surface following a fracture or in osteochondritis dissecans or synovial chondromatosis. Osteoarthritis per se does not warrant any specific treatment, but loose bodies causing locking may require removal, or the ulnar nerve may be transposed anteriorly in cases of ulnar neuritis.

3. *Flailness of the elbow*:
   The main reasons for this condition are (a) a gun shot wound, with a scar and ulnar nerve palsy, (b) Charcot's disease, where the joint can be moved painlessly in any direction and radiographs show extensive bony destruction and calcification, and (c) poliomyelitis when flailness is not a presenting symptom.
4. *Other disorders of the elbow*:

   (a) *Tennis elbow*: This is a commonly seen disorder of the elbow joint caused by minor trauma to the common extensor origin. The three main cardinal signs are (i) localized tenderness over the lateral epicondyle, (ii) pain on passive stretching and, (iii) pain on active contraction against resistance. Various forms of treatment have been tried for this condition, such as injection of the tender area with hydrocortisone and local anesthetic, physiotherapy, manipulations, rest in a sling, or lastly an operation to release the common extensor origin.
   (b) *Sports elbow*: Golfer's elbow is similar to tennis elbow, except that the flexor origin is affected. Treatment is similar. Javelin throwers may avulse the tip of the olecranon. Baseball pitchers may sustain a partial avulsion of the medial epicondyle.

5. *Loose bodies*:
   This may be due to injury, degeneration, or inflammation or be idiopathic due to synovial enchondromatosis. Clinically there are symptoms of osteoarthritis along with locking of the joint. Radiographs may show the loose body, and this can be removed when troublesome.
6. *Nerve lesions*:
   The commonest nerve to be affected is the ulnar nerve, leading to ulnar palsy. Anterior transposition of the ulnar nerve is commonly done for treatment.
7. *Bursae*:
   The olecranon bursa is most commonly affected, and it may be affected by gout, syphilis, tuberculosis, or rheumatoid arthritis. It may be excised when chronic and troublesome.

Chapter 4
Examination of the Wrist and Hand

Inspection

The attitude of the hand is noticed when the normal hand is held in slight flexion at the metacarpophalangeal and interphalangeal joints. One finger may be extended when the flexor tendon is damaged or cut in that finger. It is important to count the number of the fingers initially as it may be increased in congenital anomalies. Normal movements of the hand are smooth and synchronous. Sometimes these may be jerky and in some cases may be compensated by movements of the elbow and the shoulder joint.

The palmar surface is characterized by certain skin creases which are formed at places where the fascia attaches to the skin. The four main skin creases are as follows:

1. The distal palmar crease is located just overlying the metacarpophalangeal joints or knuckles, which also indicates the proximal edge of the surgical "no man's land," where the two flexor tendons start running in a single synovial sheath.
2. The proximal palmar crease lies at the base of the fingers and also over the proximal pulley.
3. The proximal interphalangeal crease lies at the proximal interphalangeal joints and marks the distal border of the "no man's land."
4. The thenar crease outlines the thenar group of muscles on the radial side.

The muscles are well developed, and the creases are deeper in the dominant hand as compared with the nondominant side which shows callosities. The palmar surface is actually made up of three arches: The proximal and distal arches run transversely at the carpal and metacarpal level, while the third arch runs longitudinally at its center. This area of the palm is supported by the small intrinsic muscles, and the palm loses its cup-like shape in the center when these muscles are atrophic.

The metacarpophalangeal joint on the palmar surface is characterized by "hills" and "valleys" which denote the neurovascular bundles and the place where the flexor tendons cross these joints. Normally a slight webbing is seen between the fingers, and this particularly clear between the thumb and the index fingers. This webbing may be extended into the fingers, limiting hand and finger function, as in congenital syndactyly.

K M. Iyer, *Clinical Examination in Orthopedics*,
DOI 10.1007/978-0-85729-971-0_4, © Springer-Verlag London Limited 2012

The dorsal surface is examined with the hand clenched in a fist, when the knuckle of the middle finger is the most prominent. The color of the fingernails, which are normally pink, must be carefully examined. The nails may be pale in anemia or may be spoon-shaped or split in fungal infections. Spoon-shaped or clubbed nails are commonly seen in respiratory or cardiac conditions.

Palpation

Palpation is usually done in two stages: namely, the bony elements and the soft tissue elements.

Bony Palpation

The patient's radial styloid and ulnar styloid form two basic reference points for palpation of the bony elements.

Bones of the wrist: The wrist joint is made up of two rows of carpal bones: namely, the proximal and distal rows. The proximal row from the radial to the ulnar side comprises the scaphoid, lunate, triquetrum, and pisiform which lies anterior to the triquetrum. The distal row comprises the trapezium, trapezoid, capitate, and hamate bones.

Radial styloid process: With the hand in the anatomic position, this process is lateral and has a groove with an edge at its tip.

Anatomical snuff box: This is examined just distal and dorsal to the radial styloid and is clearly seen when the thumb is extended.

Scaphoid: This is the largest bone, which forms the floor of the anatomical snuff box and is situated on the radial side of the carpus and is commonly fractured (Fig. 4.1).

It is commonly missed on initial X-rays taken of the wrist. When these X-rays are repeated after 1 week, the fracture may be clearly seen (Fig. 4.2). In clinically doubtful cases, magnetic resonance imaging is helpful in its diagnosis, particularly in medicolegal cases.

Trapezium: This is situated on the radial side of the carpus and is easily palpated when the patient flexes and extends his thumb. It is saddle shaped.

Tubercle of the radius: This is also called Lister's tubercle, and it feels like a small bony prominence which is one-third of the way across the dorsum of the wrist.

Capitate: This lies just medial to Lister's tubercle and is the largest of the carpal bones.

Lunate: This is situated in the proximal row and lies between the radius proximally and the capitate distally. The lunate, capitate, and the base of third metacarpal are located in one line, with the extensor carpi radialis brevis tendon overlying it as it inserts to the base of the third metacarpal.

Ulnar styloid process: This process does not extend as far distally as the radial styloid process. The ulnar styloid process takes no part in the wrist's articulation as

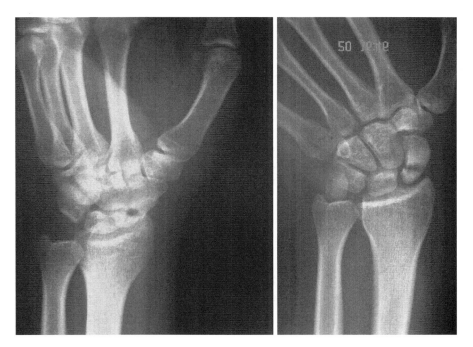

Fig. 4.1 Radiograph of fracture of the scaphoid (Courtesy Dilip Malhotra, Bahrain)

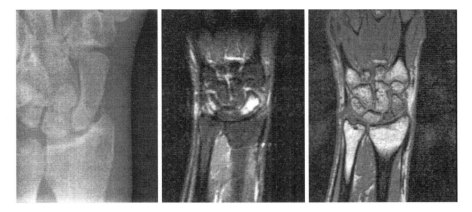

Fig. 4.2 Fracture scaphoid seen on an magnetic resonance imaging (MRI) scan 1 month after injury, which was not seen on plain X-rays taken initially (Courtesy Dushyant H. Thakkar, London, UK)

the radial side does when it articulates with the proximal row of the carpal bones. On the distal tip of the ulnar styloid process is felt a shallow groove which lodges the tendon of the extensor carpi ulnaris.

Triquetrum: The triquetrum is easily palpated as it moves out from under the styloid process when the hand is radially deviated.

Pisiform: This is a small sesamoid bone within the tendon of the flexor carpi ulnaris.

Hook of the hamate: The hook of the hamate is slightly distal and radial to the pisiform bone. This is occasionally involved in fractures, and its clinical importance lies in the fact that it forms the lateral border of Guyon's tunnel, which transports the ulnar nerve and artery into the hand, while the medial border is formed by the pisiform bone.

Metacarpals: The second and third metacarpals are relatively fixed and immobile providing stability to the index and middle fingers, as compared with the fourth and fifth metacarpals which are relatively mobile.

First metacarpal: This is palpated in continuity with the anatomical snuff box to the metacarpophalangeal joint. It is shorter and broader than the rest of the metacarpals.

Metacarpophalangeal joints: The distal palmar crease lies over the anterior aspect of the knuckles. The knuckles are palpated distally over the metacarpal ends, and their ends show a groove on the dorsal surface which lodges the long extensor tendon to the finger. Fractures of the metacarpals are common at their neck, and this is most common in the fifth metacarpal. It is known as a boxer's fracture, as it is very common in boxers (Fig. 4.3).

Phalanges: There are 14 phalanges in each hand, with the thumb having two and each of the fingers having three. The proximal interphalangeal joint is formed by the articulation of the proximal and middle phalanges, while the distal interphalangeal joint is formed by the articulation of the middle and distal phalanges. Sometimes a

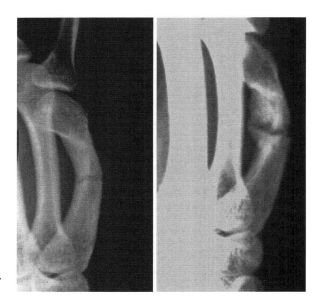

Fig. 4.3 Anteroposterior and lateral radiographs of the fifth metacarpal with no rotational deformity (Courtesy Dushyant H. Thakkar, London, UK)

callosity may be palpated over the point of a fracture due to the poor position of the fracture when it has healed.

Soft Tissue Palpation

The wrist has six tunnels for the extensor tendons and two palmar tunnels for the flexor tendons, nerves, and arteries to the hand.

Wrist Zone 1: Radial Styloid Process

The radial border of the anatomical snuff box consists of the tendons of the abductor pollicis longus and the extensor pollicis brevis, which pass over the radial styloid process. The tendon of the extensor pollicis longus passes over the ulnar border of the anatomical snuff box. The terminal branches of the superficial radial nerve are located in this interval. This forms the zone 1 of the wrist through which the tendons of the abductor pollicis longus and extensor pollicis brevis pass and are very commonly involved in stenosing tenosynovitis in de Quervain's disease. This is tested by asking the patient to make a fist with the thumb kept inside the fist and the hand deviated radially. This is known as the Finkelstein's test, and the eliciting of a sharp pain is diagnostic of this condition.

Wrist Zone II: Tubercle of the Radius

Tunnel II is on the radial side of the radial tubercle, and lodges the extensor carpi radialis longus and the extensor carpi radialis brevis. This tunnel is important as these tendons can be used in tendon transplants.

Tunnel III, which is located on the ulnar side of the radial tubercle, contains the extensor pollicis longus which takes a 45° turn around the tubercle, going to the thumb by passing over the tendons of the tunnel II – namely, the extensor carpi radialis longus and brevis. This tendon is the frequent site of rupture due to friction or rheumatoid arthritis.

Tunnel IV is situated just ulnar to tunnel III and contains the extensor digitorum communis along with the independent extensor indicis to the hand. This tunnel is frequently involved in rheumatoid arthritis and is also a frequent site for a pea-sized swelling called a ganglion, which is jelly-like in consistency and usually seen on the dorsum, and rarely on the volar, aspect of the wrist.

Wrist Zone III: Ulnar Styloid Process

This is the frequent site of pathology in a Colles' fracture or it may be involved in rheumatoid arthritis.

Tunnel V: This tunnel lodges the tendon of the extensor digiti minimi and overlies the distal ends of the dorsal radioulnar articulation on the dorsum of the wrist. The movement of the extensor digiti minimi is tested by asking the patient to raise her little finger at which point it can be felt in the depression just radial to the ulnar styloid process. Independent movement can be seen when the patient is asked to extend the index and little fingers while keeping the other fingers in a flexed position. This is popularly known as the hex sign. The abductor digiti minimi overlies the radioulnar articulation and is frequently involved in rheumatoid arthritis resulting in a rupture or may be involved in attrition from friction due to a dorsal dislocation of the ulnar head.

Tunnel VI: This is located in the groove between the ulnar styloid process and the ulnar head and contains the tendon of the extensor carpi ulnaris, which is clearly palpable when the wrist is extended and ulnarly deviated. This tendon may be involved in a Colles' fracture with an associated fracture of the distal end of the ulnar styloid process.

Wrist Zone IV: Pisiform Over the Palmar Aspect

The flexor carpi ulnaris is on the ulnar side of the palmaris longus, which has the sesamoid pisiform bone and may be the site of calcific deposits giving rise to pain.

Guyon's tunnel: This is the tunnel formed between the hook of the hamate and the pisiform bone with the overhead pisohamate ligament. It is clinically important because of passage of the ulnar nerve and artery, which may be compressed in this tunnel.

Ulnar artery: This can be palpated just proximal to the pisiform bone.

Wrist Zone V: Palmaris Longus and Carpal Tunnel

The palmaris longus stands out as a tight cord over the anterior aspect of the wrist when the patient is asked to flex the wrist and touch the tips of the thumb and little finger. It is absent in 7% of the population, and it is commonly used as a graft to replace severely injured flexor tendons of the fingers. The carpal tunnel is a tunnel beneath the palmaris longus, with its base formed by the pisiform and scaphoid in the proximal aspect, while distally it is formed by the hamate and the trapezium. The roof is formed by the transverse carpal ligament, and this tunnel transports the median nerve along with the finger flexor tendons. Compression of the carpal tunnel is a commonly seen entity which can be diagnosed by reproducing pain while tapping along the course of the median nerve over the transverse carpal ligament to elicit Tinnel's sign. Alternatively, the Phalen's test is diagnostic when tingling and numbness are reproduced by holding a flexed wrist to a maximum degree for 1 min.

Flexor carpi radialis: This is palpated by asking the patient to flex his wrist and radially deviate his hand, when the tendon stands out prominently next to the palmaris longus.

Hand Zone I: Thenar Eminence

This is situated over the base of the thumb and is made up of three muscles: namely, the abductor pollicis brevis in the superficial layer, opponens pollicis in the middle layer and flexor pollicis brevis in the deep layer. This is slightly atrophic in cases of long-standing carpal tunnel compression.

Hand Zone II: Hypothenar Eminence

This eminence is just proximal to the little finger and consists of three muscles: namely, the abductor digiti quinti, opponens digiti, and flexor digiti quinti. This eminence is supplied by the ulnar nerve, and it may be atrophied in ulnar nerve compression at Guyon's tunnel of or in the ulnar cubital tunnel.

Hand Zone III: Palm

The palmar aponeurosis consists of four divergent bands which extend to the base of the fingers. This is important clinically because it may be thickened to form discrete nodules which can cause a flexion contracture, which is commonly seen, called Dupuytren's contracture. The finger flexor tendons run in a common synovial sheath and occasionally a sudden audible click can be heard when the patient is asked to flex and extend his fingers. This is called a trigger finger when a hard nodule can be palpated in the flexor sheath just opposite the metacarpal head. A similar entity may be seen on flexing and extending the thumb, called a trigger thumb, which is commonly seen in infants.

Hand Zone IV: Dorsum

Extensor tendons: These stand out as taut chords when the patient is asked to extend his fingers while resistance is being offered. These tendons are frequently involved in rheumatoid arthritis when they are displaced to the ulnar side resulting in a classic "ulnar drift" of the fingers, which is diagnostic of rheumatoid arthritis.

Hand Zone V: Phalanges

Palpation is carried systematically starting over the proximal interphalangeal joints, which are normally smooth and may be fusiform resembling a spindle-shaped swelling. This is occasionally seen in rheumatoid arthritis and is known as Bouchard's nodes, but when seen in tuberculosis these resemble a spindle-shaped swelling called "spina ventosa." In rheumatoid arthritis, the proximal interphalangeal joint may be hyperextended with a compensatory flexion at the distal interphalangeal joint to give rise to a "swan neck deformity" of the fingers. In a reverse clinical situation, which is seen when the central slip of the extensor tendon is avulsed, the distal interphalangeal joint is hyperextended while the proximal interphalangeal joint is hyperflexed giving rise to a *boutonniere* or "button hole" deformity. Occasionally, discrete nodules may be palpable over the dorsal and lateral surfaces of the distal interphalangeal joint, which are called Heberden's nodes, and are commonly seen in osteoarthritis. In cases where the extensor tendon is avulsed at its insertion with or without a bony fragment, there may be a fixed flexion deformity of the distal interphalangeal joint called a mallet finger.

Hand Zone VI: Tufts of the Fingers

The tufts of the fingers contain terminal sensory nerve endings which are embedded in septae which when infected with pus are tense and painful. This infection may extend and enlarge the lymph nodes proximally in the supracondylar or axillary areas. A paronychia usually starts at the side of the nail and does not localize as it has room to spread around the nail base, which is commonly seen. Any infection in the finger tufts may spread along the tendon sheaths resulting in these four classic signs: The fingers are held in flexion when the fingers are swollen uniformly, there is immense pain on passive extension of the finger, and there is increased sensitivity on palpation along the course of the tendon sheaths.

Range of Motion

The movements of the wrist are mainly as follows:

1. Flexion
2. Extension
3. Radial deviation
4. Ulnar deviation
5. Supination of the forearm and
6. Pronation of the forearm.

The movements of the fingers are mainly as follows:

1. Finger flexion and extension at the metacarpophalangeal joints
2. Finger flexion and extension at the interphalangeal joints
3. Finger abduction and adduction at the metacarpophalangeal joints
4. Thumb flexion and extension at the metacarpophalangeal joint and the interphalangeal joint
5. Thumb abduction and adduction at the carpometacarpal joint and
6. Opposition.

Active Range of Motion

This is best evaluated by bilateral comparison in both wrists and hands.

1. *Wrist flexion and extension*: Normal flexion is up to 80°, and normal extension is possible up to 70°. This can be tested by asking the patient to flex and extend his wrists.
2. *Wrist ulnar and radial deviation*: This is tested by asking the patient to move his wrist sideways to ulnar and radial deviation. The radius is longer than the ulna, and hence ulnar deviation is more than radial deviation. Ulnar deviation is normally about 30°, while radial deviation is about 20°.
3. *Supination and pronation*: These tests are done as described in Chap. 3 on the elbow.
4. *Finger flexion and extension*: Ask the patient to make a fist and then extend her fingers. In normal flexion, the fingers will flex with their tips touching the distal palmar crease. Extension of the fingers is not normal if the fingers show an incomplete extension or do not extend at all.
5. *Finger abduction and adduction*: Ask the patient to spread the fingers apart and back together again. These movements are measured with the middle finger as a longitudinal axis. In abduction, the fingers should move away by 20° equally and come together in adduction of the fingers and touch each other.
6. *Thumb flexion*: Ask the patient to move his thumb across the palm and touch the base of the little finger. This movement tests for active flexion at the metacarpo-phalangeal and the interphalangeal joints of the thumb.
7. *Thumb extension*: Ask the patient to extend her thumb away from her fingers. The normal angle of thumb extension is around 50° between the index finger and the thumb.
8. *Palmar abduction and adduction of the thumb*: Ask the patient to move his thumb anteriorly from the palm and return it to the palm. Normally the range of active abduction of the thumb will be around 70° and bringing it back to the palm indicates full adduction.
9. *Opposition*: Normally the patient is able to touch the tip of the thumb to each of the other finger tips.

Passive Range of Motion

Wrist: Flexion is 80°, while extension is 70°. This can be tested passively by holding the patient's forearm in one hand and flexing and extending the wrist in the other hand. These movements are decreased in cases of ankylosis due to an infection or a malunited Colles' fracture.

Wrist: Ulnar deviation is normally 30°, while the radial deviation is 20°. These movements are decreased in cases of malunited Colles' fracture.

Fingers: Metacarpophalangeal joint flexion is normally 90°, while extension is 40°. These metacarpophalangeal joints are held by the collateral ligaments, which are slack in extension and taut in flexion, and this must be remembered when the hand is put into a cast, keeping the metacarpal joints in slight flexion to permit an easy return to normal movements with physiotherapy on removal of the cast.

Fingers: To test passive movements at the interphalangeal joints, it is very important to isolate each joint by stabilizing the phalanges proximal and distal to the joint being tested. The interphalangeal joints are equally stable in flexion and extension due to the configuration of the joint surfaces. At the proximal interphalangeal joint, flexion is normally up to 100°, while extension is 0°. At the distal interphalangeal joint, flexion is normally possible up to 90°, while extension is possible up to 20°.

Fingers: Finger abduction and adductions are purely functions of the metacarpophalangeal joints, and these are tested keeping these joints in full extension. To test this, first stabilize the metacarpal and the proximal phalanx and then move the finger into abduction and adduction.

Fingers – thumb: Thumb flexion and extension should be tested at the metacarpophalangeal and interphalangeal joints by first isolating the joints and then moving the thumb accordingly. The normal range of movement at the metacarpophalangeal joint is about 50° of flexion with extension of 0°. The interphalangeal joint normally has about 90° of flexion and 20° of extension.

Fingers – thumb: Palmar abduction and dorsal adduction are functions of the carpometacarpal joint which can be tested by first isolating this joint by stabilizing the proximal thumb and the radial styloid process. The normal range of palmar abduction possible is about 70°, and the normal range of dorsal adduction possible is nil.

Finger – opposition: Most of the movement of opposition occurs at the carpometacarpal joint of the thumb, and this is tested by holding the metacarpal of the thumb and moving it toward the palmar surface such that it touches the tips of the other fingers.

Neurologic Examination

Muscle Testing

Wrist: flexion, extension, supination, and pronation.

Fingers
– Flexion/extension
– Abduction/adduction
– Thumb flexion/extension, abduction, and adduction
– Pinch mechanism which tests the thumb and index finger
– Opposition which tests the thumb and the little finger.

Wrist Extension – C6

Primary Wrist Extensors

1. Extensor carpi radialis longus – radial nerve – C6 (C7)
2. Extensor carpi radialis brevis – radial nerve – C6 (C7)
3. Extensor carpi ulnaris – C7

   With the fingers extended, the wrist is extended slowly against gradually increasing resistance.

Wrist Flexion – C7

Primary Wrist Flexors

– Flexor carpi radialis – median nerve – C7
– Flexor carpi ulnaris – ulnar nerve – C8 (T1)

   The flexor carpi radialis is the more effective of the two wrist flexors. To test for wrist flexors, ask the patient to first make a fist which eliminates the finger flexors as wrist flexors, then stabilize the wrist by asking the patient to flex the closed fist at the wrist, and with the hand in this position, try to extend the flexed fingers.

Wrist Supination/Pronation

These are tested as described in Chap. 3 on the elbow joint.

Finger Extension – C7

Primary finger extensors are mainly three muscles:

– Extensor digitorum communis – radial nerve – C7
– Extensor indicis – radial nerve – C7 and
– Extensor digiti minimi – radial nerve – C7

   This is tested by asking the patient to extend his metacarpophalangeal joints when stabilizing the wrist in the neutral position, with the interphalangeal joints flexed which prevents finger extension being substituted by the intrinsics of the hand.

Finger Flexors – C8

Primary flexor – distal interphalangeal joint – the flexor digitorum profundus is supplied by the ulnar nerve and the anterior interosseous branch of the median nerve.

Primary flexor – proximal interphalangeal joint – the flexor digitorum superficialis is supplied by the median nerve – C7, C8, T1

Primary flexors of the metacarpophalangeal joint: These are carried out by the lumbricals, the medial two lumbricals being supplied by the ulnar nerve (C8) and the lateral two lumbricals being supplied by the median nerve (C7).

This is tested by asking the patient to flex the fingers at the interphalangeal joints and you can curl and lock your fingers into the patients fingers while trying to pull his fingers out of flexion.

Finger Abduction – T1

Primary abductors: These are the dorsal interossei which are supplied by the ulnar nerve (C8, T1) and the abductor digiti minimi which is also supplied by the ulnar nerve (C8, T1). This is tested by asking the patient to abduct his extended fingers away from the axial midline and trying to force each pair together.

Finger Adduction – T1

Primary adductors are the palmar interossei which are supplied by the ulnar nerve (C8, T1).These are tested by placing a piece of paper between two of the patient's extended fingers, in pairs.

Thumb Extension

Primary thumb extensor, metacarpophalangeal joint – extensor pollicis – brevis-radial nerve – C7

Primary thumb extensor, interphalangeal joint – radial nerve – C7

Both these joints are tested individually by asking the patient to extend his thumb, while the interphalangeal joint is tested by stabilizing the proximal phalanx of the thumb when asking the patient to extend his distal phalanx.

Thumb Flexion

Primary flexor, metacarpophalangeal joint: Thumb flexion is done by the flexor pollicis brevis and the flexor pollicis longus. The flexor pollicis brevis is supplied in its medial part by the ulnar nerve (C8), while the lateral part is supplied by the median nerve (C6, C7). The flexor pollicis longus is supplied by the median nerve (C8, T1). This is tested by asking the patient to touch his hypothenar eminence with his thumb when you are trying to pull it out of flexion.

Thumb Abduction

Primary abductors – abductor pollicis longus – radial nerve – C7
    Abductor pollicis brevis – radial nerve – C6, C7
    Test for this by first stabilizing the patient's metacarpals and then asking the patient to fully abduct his thumb against resistance.

Thumb Adduction

Primary adductor – adductor pollicis (obliquus and transversus) – ulnar nerve – C8
    Stabilize the hand and gently ask the patient to adduct her thumb against gradually increasing resistance.

Pinch Mechanism (Thumb and Index Finger)

This is a complex movement which is carried out by the long flexors and extensors which stabilize the intermetacarpal, metacarpophalangeal, and carpometacarpal joints to form a good O-type arch for pinching by the thumb and the index fingers. The lumbricals and the interossei should be functional to provide for the finger pinch motion.

Opposition (Thumb and Little Finger)

Primary opposers – opponens pollicis – median nerve – C6, C7
    Opponens digiti minimi – ulnar nerve – C8
    This is tested by asking the patient to touch the tips of his thumb and his little finger when an attempt is being done to try to pull his fingers apart.

Sensation Testing

Sensations are tested in the wrist and hand in two ways: namely, by testing the major peripheral nerves which innervate the hand and examining each neurological level in the hand.
    The three major peripheral nerves to be tested are as follows:

1. *The radial nerve*: This is tested on the web space between the thumb and the index fingers.
2. *The median nerve*: This is tested over the palmar aspect of the tip of the index finger.
3. *The ulnar nerve*: This is tested on the palmar surface of the tip of the little finger.

The sensation in the hand is supplied by three neurologic levels namely the C6 supplies sensation to the thumb, index, and half of the middle finger, while the C7 supplies sensation to the middle finger only, with contributions from C6 and C8, and the C8 supplies the ring and little fingers.

Special Tests

Long finger tests: These are mainly tests to indicate the status of the two long flexors, namely the flexor digitorum longus and the flexor digitorum superficialis.

The flexor digitorum superficialis test: Isolate the flexor digitorum superficialis by holding all of the fingers in extension except the finger being tested. Then ask the patient to flex the proximal interphalangeal joint of that finger.

Flexor digitorum profundus test: This is tested by isolating the metacarpophalangeal and the interphalangeal joints in extension and then asking the patient to flex the distal interphalangeal joint.

Bunnel-Littler test: This mainly an indication of tightness of the intrinsics (lumbricals and interossei) of the hand. It mainly helps to differentiate whether the flexion at the proximal interphalangeal joint is limited due to tightness of the intrinsics or due to contracture of the joint capsule. This test is mainly carried out by holding the metacarpophalangeal joints in a few degrees of flexion while trying to flex the proximal interphalangeal joint. If the joint can be flexed, then the intrinsics are functioning. The difference between intrinsic muscle tightness and joint capsule contracture can be seen when the finger is flexed at the metacarpophalangeal joint to relax the intrinsic and then move the interphalangeal joint into full flexion. If it can, then the intrinsics are tight, but if it cannot flex into full flexion, then it indicates a contracture of the joint capsule.

Retinacular test: This test mainly is used to note tightness of the retinacular ligaments. It is performed by holding the proximal interphalangeal joint in a neutral position and then trying to flex the distal interphalangeal joint. If the joint does not flex, then it is due to tightness of the joint capsule contracture or to retinacular tightness. At this point, flex the proximal interphalangeal joint to relax the retinaculum, then if the flexion increases at the distal interphalangeal joint, it signifies tightness of the retinacular ligaments. If the flexion does not increase, then it indicates contracture of the joint capsule of the distal interphalangeal joint.

Allen's test: This test is mainly done to test whether or not the radial and the ulnar arteries are supplying to full capacity. To test this, first ask the patient to open and close his fist several times, and thereafter occlude the radial artery with the thumb and the ulnar artery with the index and middle fingers, by compressing them against the bone. At this stage when the patient is asked to open his fist, it should be pale in color. The hand then flushes red immediately when the compressing pressure on one of the arteries is released. If the color returns only after some time, then it indicates that the artery is partially occluded.

Another version of Allen's test is as follows: Ask the patient to open and close her fist several times and with the fist still closed, place your thumb and index finger tightly on the finger to be tested for patency of the digital arteries. When the fist is opened, the finger being tested is paler than the others, while in a normal finger, the circulation returns when the pressure is released from one of the arteries.

Examination of Related Areas

In certain conditions, referred pain to the hand may be from other conditions in the upper extremity such as a ruptured cervical disc, osteoarthritis, or brachial plexus syndromes or from the shoulder and elbow. Certain specific conditions must be kept in mind when examining the wrist joint and hand.

1. *Wrist deformities*:
    (a) *Radial club hand*: Here the whole or part of the radius is absent. The wrist is palmar flexed and radially deviated, and treatment is mainly aimed toward centralizing the carpus so that it is cosmetically acceptable.
    (b) *Madelung's deformity*: This may be congenital or due to injury of the distal growth plate, where the lower radius curves forward and radially. Treatment is mainly aimed at an osteotomy of the distal radius, combined with excision of the distal ulna.
    (c) *Posttraumatic*: This is commonly seen after a Colles' fracture (Fig. 4.4).
    (d) *Postinflammation*: This may be seen in long-standing tuberculous or rheumatoid arthritis of the wrist.

2. *Stiffness of the wrist*:
    (a) *Tuberculosis*: This is usually seen when the disease has progressed. Wasting of the forearm is seen, which is obvious, and the condition is usually monoarticular. Treatment is by antituberculous drugs with a wrist splint to hold the wrist in slight dorsiflexion, and very rarely an arthrodesis is indicated.
    (b) *Kienbock's disease*: This is an avascular necrosis of the lunate. Treatment is by shortening of the radius or lengthening of the ulna in early stages. In later stages, replacement of the lunate by a silastic prosthesis or an arthrodesis of the wrist may be necessary in some cases.
    (c) *Osteoarthritis*: This is fairly uncommon and usually a sequela to minor repetitive injury. Radiographs may be helpful in some cases. Treatment is by rest in a splint, or an excision of the radial styloid process may be helpful in certain cases. Very rarely is an arthrodesis of the wrist indicated.

3. *Swellings around the wrist*:
    (a) *Ganglion*: These occur frequently on the dorsal surface of the wrist and result from a pseudomucinous degeneration of the wrist capsule or the tendon sheath which contains a viscous fluid (Fig. 4.5). When they are troublesome, the best treatment is operative excision.

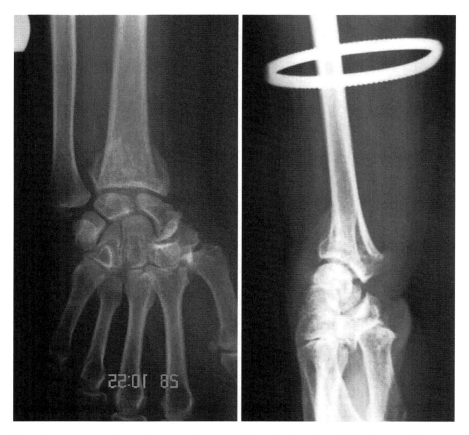

Fig. 4.4 Anteroposterior and lateral radiographs of the wrist showing a Colles' fracture (Courtesy Dilip Malhotra, Bahrain)

(b) *Compound palmar ganglion*: This is a chronic inflammation of the common flexor sheath of the flexor tendons on either sides of the flexor retinaculum of the wrist and is usually due to tuberculosis or rheumatoid arthritis. When symptomatic, the best treatment is complete excision.

(c) *Stenosing tenovaginitis*: This is also called de Quervain's disease and usually affects the tendon sheaths of the abductor pollicis longus and extensor pollicis brevis, over the radial styloid process. It usually occurs in middle-aged women and presents as a small lump which is tender. Treatment is by rest, analgesics, and injections of hydrocortisone. Should these measures not help, then an operative decompression may be necessary in some refractory cases.

4. *Deformities of the tendons*:

(a) *Mallet finger*: This is due to injury to the extensor tendon of the terminal phalanx, when the finger is held flexed at the distal interphalangeal joint with

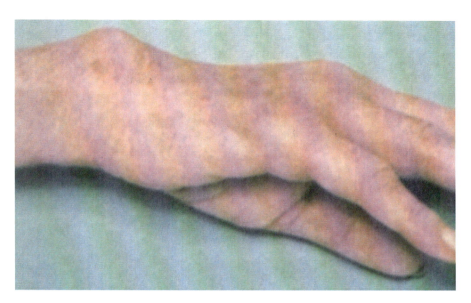

Fig. 4.5 Clinical photograph of ganglion on the dorsum of the right wrist joint (Courtesy Dilip Malhotra, Bahrain)

the patient being unable to straighten it. This is treated by a mallet splint for 6 weeks with the joint held hyperextended.

(b) *Boutonniere deformity*: This deformity follows a division of the central slip of the extensor tendon along with avulsion of the central slip near its insertion to the middle phalanx, resulting in a fixed flexion of the PIP joint along with hyperextension of the DIP joint. In established cases, this is treated by one lateral slip being transposed to the base of the middle phalanx.

(c) *Swan neck deformity*: This results from division or avulsion of the flexor digitorum sublimis tendon, when the DIP joint is held in slight flexion along with hyperextension of the PIP joint.

(d) *Tuberculous dactylitis*: This is rare, affecting only the phalanx, when there is swelling along with tenderness of a single phalanx. Treatment is by general treatment along with splintage. Should these measures not be helpful, then an amputation of the finger or ray may be considered.

(e) *Rheumatoid arthritis*: This usually causes multiple deformities in both the hands. The joints are knobby with the metacarpophalangeal joints held in flexion and the fingers deviated to the ulnar side.

(f) *Gout*: This may involve both hands and the characteristic tophi may be seen.

5. *Other deformities*: Dupuytren's contracture:
This is a disease which is confined to individuals of European descent and is commonly associated with epilepsy, alcoholic cirrhosis, and pulmonary tuberculosis. Most of the patients are men, and it affects the palmar fascia of both hands, most commonly opposite the ring finger (Fig. 4.6).

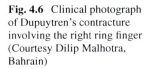
Fig. 4.6 Clinical photograph
of Dupuytren's contracture
involving the right ring finger
(Courtesy Dilip Malhotra,
Bahrain)

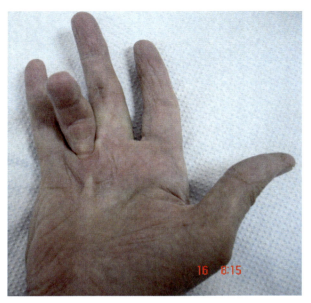

The palmar fascia thickens and shrinks, with the finger being pulled into gradual flexion. When this condition is gradually increasing and becoming a nuisance, operations such as a fasciotomy or fasciectomy may be carried out, before resorting to more radical measures such as amputation of the finger when severely affected.

6. *Tunnel syndromes*:

   (a) *Carpal tunnel syndrome*: This syndrome is seen in menopausal women, rheumatoid arthritis and pregnancy, when there is insufficient space for the median nerve to travel beneath the transverse carpal ligament. This results in paresthesia and numbness along the distribution of the median nerve in the hand. Tinnel's sign is positive, and the sensory changes can be reproduced by holding the wrist palmar flexed for 1 min. The diagnosis can also be confirmed on electromyography. This is treated initially conservatively by an injection of hydrocortisone into the flexor sheath or by wearing a cock-up wrist splint. Refractory cases are best treated by decompression involving the division of the transverse carpal ligament of the wrist joint.

   (b) *Stenosing tenovaginitis of the flexor tendons*: This is seen when there is insufficient space for normal tendon action, or may be seen in rheumatoid arthritis or due to thickening of the fibrous sheath or to a nodular thickening of the tendon. Any finger may be thus affected, which results in a tender area when the patient bends the affected finger, followed by clicking of the affected finger, which is painful. It may be seen in infants as a small hard nodule, which is commonly seen in the thumb. Treatment is usually by a small transverse incision whereby the fibrous sheath is incised and decompressed until the tendon moves freely.

Fig. 4.7 Clinical photograph of
paronychia (Courtesy of Shabih
Siddiqui, Kettering, UK)

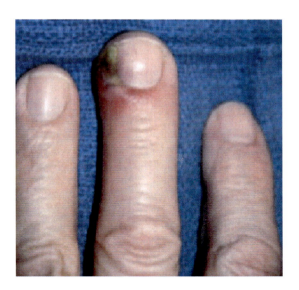

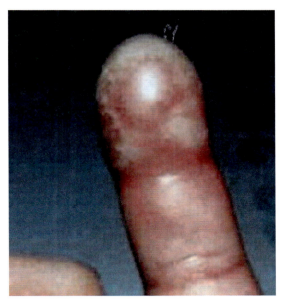

Fig. 4.8 Clinical photograph of
pulp infection (Courtesy of Shabih
Siddiqui, Kettering, UK)

7. *Acute infections of the hand*:

    (a) *Paronychia*: Acute infections at the base of the nail are very common. The
infected area is reddish and warm. Treatment is by excision of a part of the
nail along with appropriate antibiotics (Fig. 4.7).

    (b) *Whitlow*: Pulp infection is fairly common and early drainage is essential
under antibiotic prophylaxis (Fig. 4.8).

(c) *Suppurative tenosynovitis*: Infection of tendon sheath is uncommon and painful. The middle three fingers may be involved, or the thumb and the little finger may be involved alone. The affected finger is swollen and looks like a sausage. Treatment is by adequate drainage of the synovial sheath by incisions near their proximal or distal ends or both.

(d) *Infection of the fascial spaces*: This may result from spread of the infection from a web space or the tendon sheath to the deep fascial spaces of the palm. Hence it may spread to the midpalmar or the thenar space as the case may be. It is treated by adequate drainage under antibiotic prophylaxis.

8. *Open injuries of the hand*:

(a) *Primary treatment*: This includes a thorough cleaning with antibiotic prophylaxis, along with wound excision, and deep repair along with primary wound closure wherever possible. Postoperatively, the hand is kept elevated and the dressings are taken off at 3 weeks, when an assessment can be done with accuracy. Further rehabilitation may be started when the primary wounds have healed.

(b) *Secondary operations*: This may be necessary in the form of secondary repair of the damaged structures, amputation of the fingers, or a reconstruction of the mutilated hand, which are best dealt with by a hand expert.

Chapter 5
Examination of the Hip and Pelvis

The pelvic girdle is formed by three main joints: namely, the hip joints, sacroiliac joints, and symphysis pubis.

Inspection

This is done as the patient enters the examining room and the patient has completely removed his clothes to make this inspection quite simple. Observe for any abrasions, discolourations, birth marks, sinuses, and scars and any swellings. Also observe the patient's gait and stance to see if both the anterior superior iliac spines are on the same horizontal plane, and some impression may be had by this observation for any tilted pelvis due to limb length discrepancy. An inspection may also be made from the side, which gives an idea of the normal lumbar lordosis which is seen. Absence of this may be seen in cases of spasm of the paravertebral muscles in disc pathology.

An inspection is also carried out from the posterior aspect to see if the two gluteal folds are symmetrical on both sides. In infants, asymmetrical folds may be seen in congenital dislocation of the hip, muscular dystrophy, or limb length discrepancy. When viewed from the posterior aspect, two dimples are also seen which overlie the posterior superior iliac spines just above the buttocks.

Palpation

Bony palpation is carried out anteriorly and posteriorly.

K M. Iyer, *Clinical Examination in Orthopedics*,
DOI 10.1007/978-0-85729-971-0_5, © Springer-Verlag London Limited 2012

Anterior Aspect

Anterior superior iliac spines: In most patients, these bony prominences are subcutaneous, being palpated on the sides of the waist.

Iliac crest: The Iliac crest is subcutaneous in most of its course, and both the crests are level with each other.

Iliac tubercle: This is felt as a bony prominence on the outer wall of the iliac crest when palpating posteriorly along the iliac crest.

Greater trochanter: These can be palpated by the hand moving down from the iliac tubercles. Normally both the trochanters are on the same horizontal level, but this relation is disturbed in cases of congenital dislocation of the hip or a fracture of the hip.

Pubic tubercles: Palpation is then continued medially toward the midline where the pubic tubercles can be felt as bony prominences under the pubic hair.

Posterior Aspect

This is best examined with the patient lying on his side.

Posterior superior iliac spines: These are easily palpable over the dimples which are just above the buttocks. The spines are easily palpable and subcutaneous in nature.

Greater trochanter: Palpating downwards from the posterior superior iliac spine, the posterior border of the greater trochanter can be felt.

Ischial tuberosity: This is easily palpated when the hips are flexed, when the gluteus maximus moves upwards and the ischial tuberosity is felt. Both the tuberosities lie on the same horizontal plane as the lesser trochanters.

Sacroiliac joint: This joint is not usually palpable, because of the overhanging ilium and its ligaments.

Soft tissue palpation is carried out in five zones:

Zone I: Femoral Triangle

The femoral triangle has its base at the inguinal ligament which extends between the anterior superior iliac spines and the pubic tubercles. Any unusual bulges seen and felt along this may indicate an inguinal hernia. The femoral artery is normally felt as a strong pulse beneath the midway point of the anterior superior iliac spine and the pubic tubercle. Just beneath the femoral artery is the femoral head. The femoral nerve lies just lateral to the artery though it is not palpable. The femoral vein lies just medial to the artery and is a common site for venous puncture.

Sartorius muscle: This is the longest muscle in the body and forms the lateral border of the femoral triangle. It is usually palpable at its origin just inferior to the anterior superior iliac spine.

Adductor longus muscle: This muscle can be palpated as a distinct ridge when the legs are abducted. In spastic children, this muscle may be tenotomized to release the limb from severe adduction and thus prevent dislocation of the hip.

The femoral triangle is palpated for lymph nodes which may be enlarged in infection from the lower limb or the pelvis. These are usually located most medially in the femoral triangle.

Zone II

This mainly consists of the greater trochanter and the gluteus medius muscle.

Greater trochanter: Palpate the greater trochanter for any tenderness, and usually a bursa is felt over the bone as a boggy swelling.

The gluteus medius muscle is usually inserted into the lateral part of the greater trochanter. Occasionally when the hip is flexed and adducted, the tensor fascia lata may ride anteriorly over the greater trochanter and may give an audible click when it returns to the neutral position.

Zone III: Sciatic Nerve

This is located exactly midway between the greater trochanter and the ischial tuberosity. This is covered by the gluteus maximus with the hip in extension, which moves away when the hip is flexed. Tenderness over the nerve may be seen in a herniated lumbar disc, spasm of the piriformis, or in cases of direct trauma over the nerve as in nerve injections. Similarly the bursa covering the ischial tuberosity may be inflamed giving rise to ischial bursitis.

Zone IV: Iliac Crest

The cluneal nerves supply the skin over the iliac crest between the posterior superior iliac spines and the tubercles, and these are cut when taking a bone graft. Therefore this area should be palpated for any neuromas in the cluneal nerves.

Zone V: Hip and Pelvic Muscles

These are mainly arranged in four quadrants: namely, (1) flexor group – anterior quadrant, (2) abductor grouping – lateral quadrant, (3) adductor grouping – medial quadrant and (4) extensor grouping – posterior quadrant.

1. *Flexor grouping*: The Iliopsoas muscle is primarily a hip flexor. The iliopsoas bursa lies deep beneath the muscle, and infection may result in a painful iliopsoas bursitis.
   Sartorius muscle: This is a long strap-like muscle which runs along the anterior aspect of the thigh.
   Rectus femoris: This muscle crosses the hip and the knee joints, thereby acting as a flexor of the hip and an extensor of the knee. This muscle has its origin in two heads, and both these heads may be pulled or torn from their heads in sports injuries.
2. *Adductor grouping*: This group is formed by five muscles: namely, the gracilis, pectineus, adductor longus, adductor brevis, and the adductor magnus. Of these muscles, the adductor longus is the most superficial and can be palpated.
3. *Abductor grouping*: This group consists of two main muscles: namely, the gluteus medius and the gluteus minimus. Of these, the gluteus minimus lies deep under the gluteus medius and is therefore not palpable. The gluteus medius is the main hip abductor and is palpable at its insertion along the anterior and lateral aspects of the greater trochanter. Weakness of this muscle results in a characteristic "gluteus medius lurch."
4. *Extensor grouping*: This mainly consists of the gluteus maximus and the hamstrings. The gluteus maximus is easily palpable when the patient is lying prone with hip extended and buttocks squeezed together. The hamstring muscles consist of the biceps femoris on the lateral side with the semitendinosus and the semimembranosus on the medial side. Generalized spasm of the hamstrings ("pulled hamstring") is commonly seen after athletic activity or may be seen in spondylolisthesis or a herniated lumbar spinal disc.

Range of Motion

Active Range of Movements

1. *Abduction*: This is tested by asking the patient to stand and spread his legs wide apart. The normal range possible is around 45°.
2. *Adduction*: This is tested by asking the patient to cross his legs and should be about 20°.
3. *Flexion*: This is tested by asking the patient to flex his hips toward the chest, and this should be around 135°.
4. *Flexion and adduction*: This is tested by asking the patient to sit on a chair and cross one thigh over the other.
5. *Flexion, abduction, and external rotation*: This is tested by asking the patient to place the lateral side of his foot on his opposite knee.
6. *Extension*: This is tested by asking the patient to get up from the sitting position with his back straight and his arms across his chest.
7. *Internal and external rotation*: These are tested by the patient lying supine and prone.

Passive Range of Movements

Flexion (Thomas') test: This is a specific test designed to assess flexion contracture of the hip joint in addition of the range of flexion in the hip joint. Test the flexion as flexing the hip on the patients chest to see if it is possible to touch the thigh to the chest. When the knee is at the chest wall, have the patient hold this limb with his hand and allow the other limb to fall straight onto the examining table. If this not fully possible, then the patient has a fixed flexion contracture of that hip.

Extension: This is tested by asking the patient to lie prone. The pelvis and hip are stabilized with one hand on the pelvis while the other hand flexes the knee to relax the hamstrings. Then the hip extension is tested by extending the thigh, which should extend to around 30°.

Abduction: This is tested with the patient lying supine and the pelvis stabilized at the iliac crests. The lower limb is held at the ankle and abducted in one piece, normally to around 45°. This is more often limited by pathology than adduction.

Adduction: This is tested by continuing above maneuver from full abduction until the limb returns back to the normal position, which is normally around 30°.

Internal/external rotation: These are tested in two ways: with the hips flexed and extended. In the first approach, with the patient lying supine, both limbs are held just above the malleoli and rotated to examine the angle at which the patella faces. The normal angle of internal rotation is 30°, while the normal angle of external rotation is 45°. In the other approach, keeping the patient supine, let his legs hang down from his flexed knees. In this position the tibia is the pendulum which measures the angles of internal and external rotation at the hip joints.

Yet another method to test these movements with the patient supine and the knees extended is to observe the upward direction of both big toes, which can be used as a marker for these angles. This also takes into account the normal angle of anteversion at the neck of the femur, when the patient is lying flat. Any decrease in the angle of internal rotation may lead one to suspect a slipped upper femoral epiphysis in the growing child. In an adult, osteoarthritis may cause limitation to these movements, though internal rotation is more frequently limited in that condition.

Neurologic Examination

Muscle Testing

Flexors

Primary flexor: iliopsoas – femoral nerve – L1, L2, L3
Secondary flexor: rectus femoris

This is tested by the patient sitting at the edge of the table with her legs hanging over the edge. The patient is asked to raise her thigh against gradually increasing resistance (Table 5.1).

Table 5.1 Muscle grading chart

Muscle gradations	Description
5 – Normal	Complete range of motion against gravity with full resistance
4 – Good	Complete range of motion against gravity with some resistance
3 – Fair	Complete range of motion against gravity
2 – Poor	Complete range of motion against with gravity eliminated
1 – Trace	Evidence of slight contractility. No joint motion
0 – Zero	No evidence of contractility

Extensors

Primary extensor: gluteus maximus – inferior gluteal nerve – S1
Secondary extensor: hamstrings
   This is tested with the patient lying prone with the leg flexed at the knee to relax the hamstrings. The patient is asked to extend his thigh during this maneuver.

Abductors

Primary abductor: gluteus medius – superior gluteal nerve – L5
   Secondary abductor: gluteus minimus
   This is tested by the patient lying on his side. The patient is asked to abduct her leg. Alternatively, this can be tested by the patient lying supine, with the legs abducted against gradually increasing resistance.

Adductors

Primary adductor: adductor longus – obturator nerve – L2, L3, L4
Secondary adductors: adductor brevis, adductor magnus, pectineus, and gracilis.
   In continuation with the above test, this test is carried out by placing the hand over the medial side of the thigh. The patient is asked to pull her limb back toward the midline, or alternatively the patient may be asked to adduct her legs with gradually increasing resistance over the medial aspect of the knees.

Sensation Testing

The dermatomes of the anterior abdominal wall run in oblique bands, with the umbilicus being supplied by the T10 dermatome. The strip just above the inguinal ligament is supplied by the T12 dermatome, and the area in between this and the umbilicus is supplied by the T11 dermatome. The dermatome just below the inguinal ligament is supplied by the L1, while the dermatome just above the knee joint is supplied by the L3. The area in between these two regions is supplied by the L2 dermatome.

The posterior primary divisions of the cluneal nerves L1, L2, and L3 cross over the posterior iliac crest and supply sensation to (1) the area just over the iliac crest, (2) the area between the posterior superior iliac spine and the iliac tubercle and (3) the area over both the buttocks. The posterior cutaneous nerve of the thigh (S2) supplies a longitudinal area along the posterior aspect of the thigh, while the lateral cutaneous nerve (S3) of the thigh supplies a broad area over the lateral aspect of the thigh. The dermatomes around the anus are arranged in three concentric rings with the innermost being supplied by S1 and the outermost being the S3, while the S2 supplies the intermediate ring.

Special Tests

Trendelenburg's test: This test is completed by examining the level of the iliac crests from behind when the patient stands and bears weight on one leg. This tests the gluteus medius muscle which can be seen to be affected if there is a drop in the level of the iliac crest on the affected side. This test can also be positive when it is delayed up to 1 min by an insufficiency of the gluteus medius muscle. Numerous conditions can give rise to a weak gluteus medius muscle, such as a slipped upper femoral epiphysis, congenital dislocation of the hip or certain neurologic conditions such as poliomyelitis or a meningomyelocele.

Limb length discrepancy: If on inspection, one suspects a limb length discrepancy, then actual measurements of the limbs can determine this feature.

True limb length discrepancy: This is tested by placing both the lower limbs in identical positions with both the iliac crests parallel, and measuring the lengths between anterior superior iliac spines and the medial malleoli. To determine whether the discrepancy is in the tibia or the femur, ask the patient to lie flat with the knees flexed to 90° and the heels flat on the examining table. When the level of the knees are seen to be lower, then it is the femur that is shorter, as in poliomyelitis or in case of a malunited fracture.

Apparent limb length discrepancy: This is noticed in cases where there is pelvic obliquity or in cases of an adduction contracture of the hip joint. This is examined by asking the patient to lie supine with his lower limbs in the neutral position. The distance is then measured from the umbilicus to the medial malleolus of the ankle.

Ober's test: This test is mainly done for a contraction of the iliotibial band. Ask the patient to lie on her side with the involved side being uppermost. Abduct the leg as far as possible and flex the knee to 90° to relax the iliotibial band, allowing the involved limb to drop down to the adducted position. Continued abduction of the leg indicates an abduction contracture of the iliotibial band. This may be seen in poliomyelitis or a meningomyelocele.

Test for congenital dislocation of the hip:

1. *Ortolani click*: This test is completed by flexing the hip along with abduction, and externally rotating it. It can be felt to slip out of the hip joint to be reduced back into the joint during adduction and internal rotation with an audible click. In cases of congenital dislocation of the hip, abduction is markedly limited in itself.

2. *Telescoping*: This is tested by stabilizing the pelvis with one hand, while the other hand pushes and pulls the femur. Telescoping is felt as a to-and-fro movement of the greater trochanter.
3. *Adduction contracture*: This is tested by abducting a flexed hip. Abduction is not possible in an adduction contracture of the hip joint. Normally abduction should be possible in a flexed hip up to about 90°.

Examination of Related Areas

The hip and pelvis examination is completed with a proper rectal examination. While testing, the gloved finger first examines the superficial anal reflex (S2, S3, S4) to touch. While doing a rectal examination, palpate the inner surface of the rectal wall which should be smooth and not fixed and immobile. During palpation, the internal sphincter is felt to grip your finger in a contraction which is the deep anal reflex (S5). Also the prostatic groove can be palpated clearly before proceeding to palpate the sacroiliac joint and the bony coccyx which is normally mobile in bimanual palpation.

Certain conditions which are very specific must always be kept in mind:

1. *Congenital dislocation of the hip*: This is a condition which can be diagnosed early in life, and various tests are very helpful in its diagnosis in addition to early radiographs (Figs. 5.1 and 5.2). A hip with a positive Barlow's or Ortolani sign may become normal with time, without any treatment. Treatment before weight bearing consists of an abduction napkin or a Von Rosen splint. Treatment after weight bearing is by gradually increasing vertical traction, followed by a plaster or a Dennis Brown splint. Surgical treatment is considered when the closed treatment fails, and an open reduction is considered with or without a Salter's osteotomy or derotation osteotomy to keep the reduction stable.

   (a) *Subluxation of the hip*: This is commonly seen in acetabular dysplasia, when the femoral head is not displaced but subluxated upwards over the innominate bone. Radiographs taken at this stage are diagnostic. Treatment is by traction and a Dennis Brown splint to be worn until the acetabular roof looks normal. In older children, surgical treatment is directed toward providing a good acetabular roof by a Salter's innominate osteotomy or Chiari's pelvic osteotomy, or by constructing a massive shelf.

   (b) *Pathological dislocation of the hip*: This may result from early pyogenic arthritis giving rise to a dislocation, and radiographs are diagnostic. This is usually treated by aspiration under anesthesia, along with systemic antibiotics and a Dennis Brown splint for 3 months.

   (c) *The irritable hip*: This is usually seen in nonspecific synovitis with pain and limp. Treatment is by bed rest with traction and analgesics. Blood investigations help in establishing the diagnosis, and certain conditions such as transient synovitis, tuberculosis, chronic synovitis, Perthes' disease, and slipped upper femoral epiphysis must be considered in the differential diagnosis.

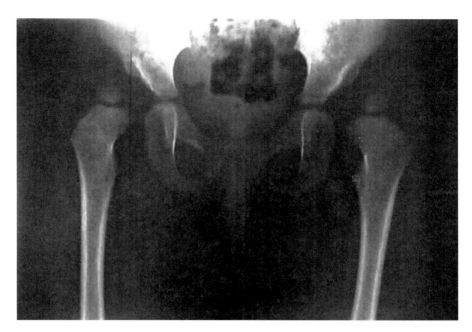

Fig. 5.1 Anteroposterior radiograph of the pelvis with both hips showing bilateral congenital dislocation of the hip (Courtesy Dilip Malhotra, Bahrain)

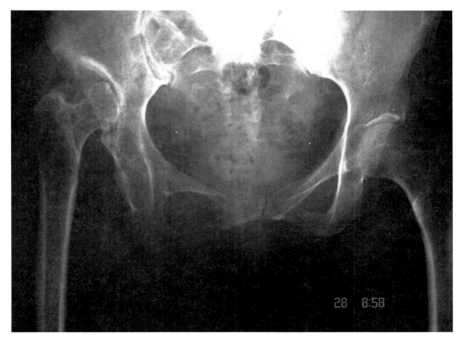

Fig. 5.2 Anteroposterior radiograph of the pelvis with both hips showing a neglected congenital dislocation of the right hip (Courtesy Dilip Malhotra, Bahrain)

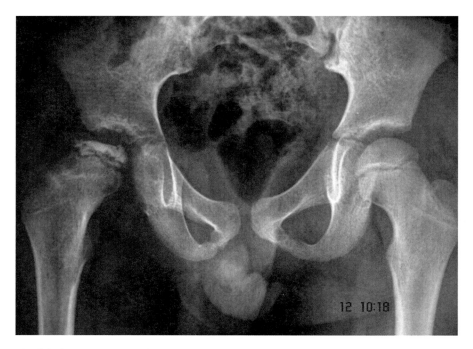

Fig. 5.3 Anteroposterior radiograph of the pelvis showing early Perthes' disease of the right hip (Courtesy Dilip Malhotra, Bahrain)

2. *Tuberculosis of the hip*: This usually starts as a synovitis, and destruction of the hip is very rapid with muscle spasm and wasting. Healing leaves an unsound hip with fibrous ankylosis characterized by limb shortening and deformity. Secondary infection may occur, with the development of bony ankylosis. Initial treatment is by antituberculous drugs with traction. Later on surgical treatment is by an osteotomy or arthrodesis or a combination of both.

3. *Perthes' disease*: This is a condition seen in the first few years of life due to partly or wholly avascular necrosis of the head of the femur (Fig. 5.3). Gradually this dead head is replaced by creeping substitution, resulting in revascularization of the femoral head along with varying degrees of flattening and coxa vara. The various stages of the disease are clearly recognizable on serial radiographs. Treatment is by traction, avoiding weight bearing, and containment of the femoral head within the acetabulum (Fig. 5.4).

4. *Slipped upper femoral epiphysis*: This condition may be seen due to trauma, and sometimes an underlying abnormality is strongly suggested such as an endocrine imbalance. In the majority of the cases, it is bilateral, though unilateral cases are also known in about 30% of cases. Clinically, the limb shows diminished abduction along with medial rotation and an increased lateral rotation. Radiographs are diagnostic by Trethovan's and Capener's signs, and indications on lateral radiographs are very obvious from the very start of the

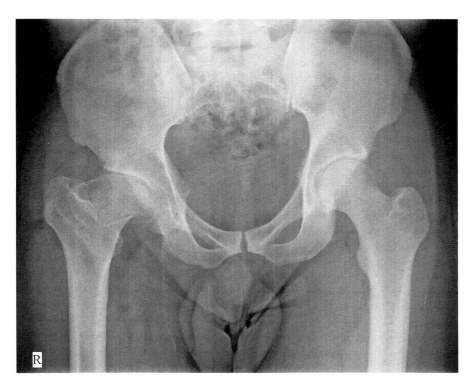

Fig. 5.4 Anteroposterior radiograph showing an old, healed Perthes' disease of the right hip (Courtesy Dilip Malhotra, Bahrain)

condition (Fig. 5.5). Treatment is by fixing the displaced femoral head in situ with multiple pinning without any attempt at reduction. In some cases a geometric fixation osteotomy or subtrochanteric osteotomy is carried out to correct the deformity in order to make the growth plate more horizontal.

5. *Coxa vara*: Here the neck shaft angle is reduced. This may be congenital or acquired. Radiographs may be helpful in some cases when a separate triangular piece of bone may be seen in the inferior part of the metaphysis. This is usually treated by a corrective subtrochanteric osteotomy.

6. *Osteoarthritis*: This is a condition where the articular cartilage is worn away in pressure areas, while in nonpressure areas, the cartilage may become dense and thicker, giving rise to osteophytes and lipping. Concurrent synovial hypertrophy also occurs, and clinically the condition is diagnosed by rest pain at night along with decreased painful movements of the hip in its extreme degrees. There is obvious shortening of the limb with elevation of the greater trochanter, and radiographs are very helpful in its diagnosis. Initial treatment is usually conservative in the form of heat, manipulation, and an injection of hydrocortisone. Eventually surgical treatment is indicated, including any of three main operations: namely, osteotomy, arthrodesis arthroplasty. A McMurray's

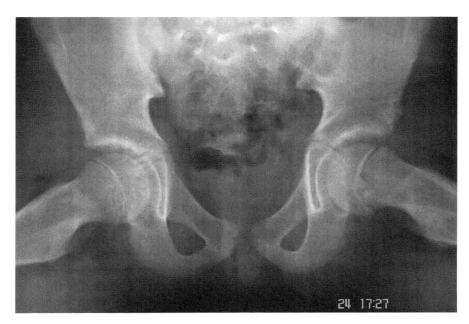

Fig. 5.5 Anteroposterior radiograph of the pelvis taken in frog's view showing a slipped upper femoral epiphysis on the left side (Courtesy Dilip Malhotra, Bahrain)

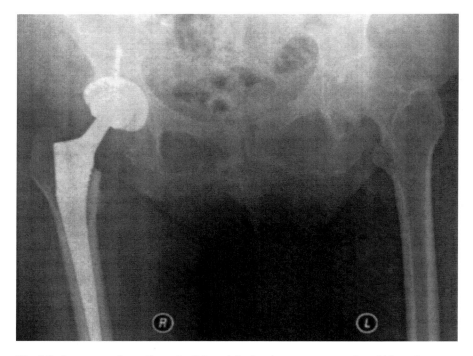

Fig. 5.6 Anteroposterior radiograph of the pelvis showing an uncemented total hip replacement of the right hip (Courtesy Dushyant H. Thakkar, London, UK)

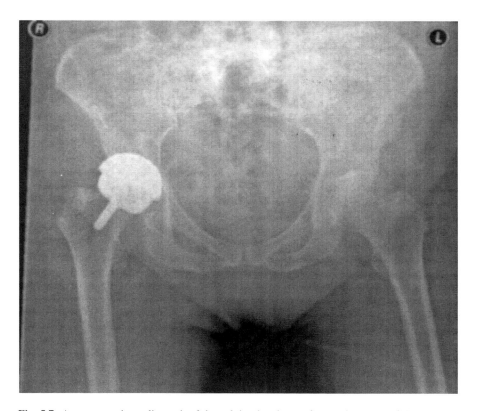

Fig. 5.7 Anteroposterior radiograph of the pelvis, showing surface replacement of the right hip (Courtesy Dushyant H. Thakkar, London, UK)

displacement osteotomy is valuable in the early stages if the disease is segmental: The femur is divided in the subtrochanteric region, and the displacement fixed by means of a compression plate. Arthrodesis is a certain way of achieving a pain-free joint, but this has been discarded these days with the evolution in arthroplasty. With the advent of total joint arthroplasty, Girdlestone's arthroplasty of an excision of the hip joint has been reserved as a salvage operation for failed cases of total joint arthroplasty. Total hip arthroplasty or low friction arthroplasty was revolutionized by Charnley five decades ago. Nowadays, uncemented total hip replacement is in vogue, because of the shorter operating time involved, avoiding the complications postoperatively of using bone cement (Fig. 5.6). Another form of arthroplasty which is done nowadays is surface replacement of the femoral head (Fig. 5.7), whereby an excision of the femoral head is avoided as is done in a total hip arthroplasty. The latter can be reserved for any future salvage operations, such as revision of the surface replacement by its conversion to a total hip arthroplasty.

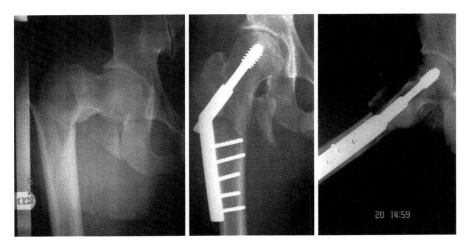

Fig. 5.8 Radiographs show an extracapsular (intertrochanteric) fracture of the right hip, which has been treated by a sliding dynamic compression hip screw and plate (Courtesy Dilip Malhotra, Bahrain)

7. *Fracture neck of femur*: This is a very common condition and is frequently seen in the elderly. In the past, it was well known "to be the beginning of the end." Considerable interest still prevails in this condition, and it is now called "the unsolved fracture." The most important point to note is whether the fracture is intracapsular or extracapsular. It is imperative for it to be diagnosed as early as possible, so that necessary treatment can be started as early as possible. Various forms of treatment have been tried in the past, and it has been universally agreed that these fractures should be treated as early as possible. The basic aim for early treatment is to put the patient on their feet again as soon as possible (Figs. 5.8–5.10).

8. *Avascular necrosis of the hip*: This is a condition which must be kept in mind for differential diagnosis where an early decrease in rotations of the hip joint are seen (Fig. 5.11). It results in an area of avascularity of a segment of the hip, and the patient complains of pain only. It may be bilateral in alcoholics. This condition may also be seen in liver disorders or may be seen as an idiopathic variety.

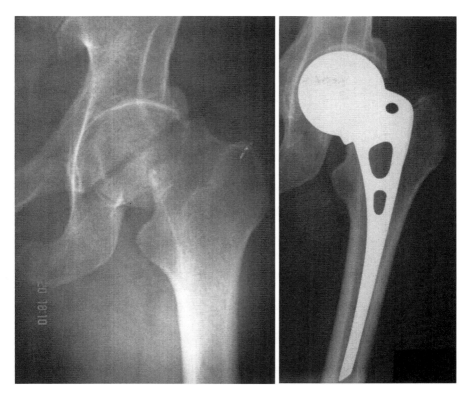

Fig. 5.9 Radiographs showing a displaced intracapsular fracture (transcervical) of the left hip which has been treated by an Austin Moore prosthesis (Courtesy Dilip Malhotra, Bahrain)

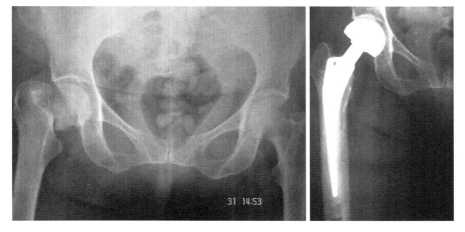

Fig. 5.10 Radiographs showing a displaced intracapsular fracture (transcervical) of the right hip treated by a cemented bipolar prosthesis (Courtesy Dilip Malhotra, Bahrain)

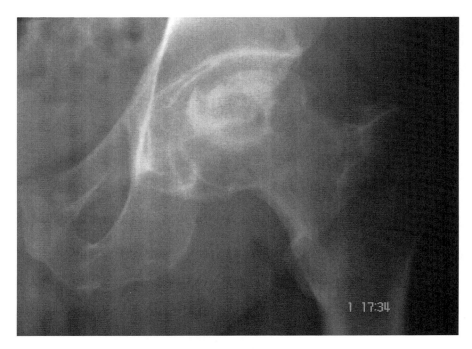

Fig. 5.11 Anteroposterior radiograph of the left hip joint showing avascular necrosis of the weight-bearing segment of the femoral head (Courtesy Dilip Malhotra, Bahrain)

Chapter 6
Examination of the Knee

The knee is the largest modified hinge joint in the body, which provides the greatest range of movement in flexion of the joint.

Inspection

Inspect the patient's gait while asking him to undress to expose the knee joints. Examine the patient standing up, when the normal knee has a slight degree of valgus in the leg with respect to the femur. An increase in this angle is called genu valgum, and it results in both the knees touching one another to produce a knock knee. Obliteration of the normal valgus ankle results in a genu varum called bow legs. When seen sideways, the knee joint is extended, which can be exaggerated, and this may be bilateral, as in females due to hyperlaxity of ligaments resulting in a genu recurvatum. Inspect the quadriceps muscles just above the knee joint. These may be decreased in size or atrophied following knee surgery. Intra-articular hemorrhage and synovitis with synovial thickening may be seen as a generalized swelling which obliterates the normal contour of the knee joint.

Above all, look for any localized swellings around the knee. A bursal swelling is commonly seen in front of the patella and is known as a prepatellar bursitis, or it may be seen inferiorly over the tibial tubercle, which is known as an infrapatellar bursitis. Occasionally a localized swelling may be seen in the popliteal fossa, such as a Baker's cyst, or it may be located just over the medial aspect of the tibial tubercle, which is known as a pes anserinus bursa.

K M. Iyer, *Clinical Examination in Orthopedics*,
DOI 10.1007/978-0-85729-971-0_6, © Springer-Verlag London Limited 2012

Palpation

The bony components of the knee joint are best palpated with the knee in slight flexion as they all disappear in full extension of the knee. Furthermore, the muscles, tendons, and ligaments are lax in the flexed non-weight-bearing position, thus facilitating examination of the bony landmarks and joint margins.

Medial Aspect

This is best palpated by the thumbs over the joint line.

Medial tibial plateau: Move your thumb just inferiorly, and the sharp ridge of the medial tibial plateau can be palpated, which is also the attachment of the medial meniscus.

Tibial tubercle: Continue with the inspecting finger inferiorly until it reaches the bony tibial tubercle. The area just medial to this is of importance as the insertion to the tendon of the pes anserinus and the bursa.

Medial femoral condyle: This is palpated just medial to the patella, and a greater area can be palpated by increasing knee flexion to more than 90°. Sometimes a bony defect may be palpated in cases of osteochondritis dissecans. Osteophytes may be palpated at the edges of patients with osteoarthritis.

Adductor tubercle: This can be identified by proceeding upward and posteriorly up the medial femoral condyle, in the distal part of the natural depression between the vastus medialis and the hamstrings.

Lateral Aspect

Lateral tibial plateau: This is a sharp ridge just between the junction of the tibia and the femur.

Lateral tubercle: This is a large bony prominence immediately below the lateral tibial plateau.

Lateral femoral condyle: More of the articulating articular surface is palpable with the knee flexed more than 90°, as the finger moves upward. The amount of the lateral femoral condyle available for palpation is much less than the medial femoral condyle because most of the surface of the lateral femoral condyle is covered by the patella.

Lateral femoral epicondyle: This lies just lateral to the lateral femoral condyle.

Head of the fibula: Proceeding with palpation slightly inferiorly and posteriorly along the joint line, the fibular head is palpated at the same level as the tibial tuberosity.

Trochlear Groove and Patella

The trochlear groove is the path along which the patella tracks, and it can be palpated by both thumbs along the medial and lateral joint lines to the highest point of the patella – just above that is a depression of the trochlear groove. The patella is fixed in flexion of the knee joint and is mobile in full extension, when it is easier to push the patella to the medial side than the lateral side.

Soft Tissue Palpation

This is carried out in the following four zones: anterior, medial, lateral, and posterior.

Zone I: Anterior Aspect

Quadriceps: This is a massive muscle which is formed of three parts – the medialis, intermedius, and lateralis – and together with the rectus femoris, it forms a common tendon inserting into the superior and medial borders of the patella and carrying on as the infrapatellar tendon to be finally inserted into the tibial tubercle. The muscle mass of the medialis extends further distally than the lateralis. Observe for any defects just proximal to the patella. These may be seen in ruptures which are transverse in nature. Signs of atrophy may be seen in the vastus medialis frequently following knee surgery or an effusion. The actual measurements of atrophy of the quadriceps muscle may be taken at similar points in both the thighs, with the tibial tubercle or the tibial plateau being taken as reference points for this.

Infrapatellar tendon: This is inserted into the tibial tubercle which may be tender in children, in which case it is called Osgood–Schlatter's syndrome. The infrapatellar tendon may be avulsed from its insertion, when it does not feel rigid and a palpable defect can be felt. The infrapatellar region is palpated for any signs of bursitis, which is fairly common. These bursae are mainly located in the anterior aspect of the knee joint and they may be superficial or deep to the patellar tendon. The superficial infrapatellar bursa lies between the patellar tendon and the skin and may become inflamed with constant kneeling.

Another common site is the tendon of the pes anserinus where the bursa lies just beneath the tendon of the pes anserinus. This is known as the pes anserine bursa. The prepatellar bursa is located just over the anterior part of the patella, and it may be involved after constant kneeling in what is referred to as "housemaid's knee."

Zone II: Medial Aspect

Medial meniscus: This is located just above the medial tibial plateau and is anchored by coronary ligaments. It may be tender when involved in tears. The medial meniscus is mobile as compared with the lateral meniscus. When the tibia is rotated externally the anterior margin of the medial meniscus is palpable in the joint space. Tears of the medial meniscus are more frequent than tears of the lateral meniscus.

Medial collateral ligament: This is a broad fan-shaped ligament which has two portions and lies between the medial femoral condyle and the upper tibia. The deep part extends to the edge of the upper tibial plateau and the medial meniscus, while the superficial part extends more distally over the flare of the upper tibia. This medial collateral ligament is intimately blended with the joint capsule and is frequently torn in valgus injuries, as seen in football. In cases of avulsion from the medial epicondyle, a small chip of the bone may be taken with the ligament when the point of origin is tender on palpation.

Sartorius, gracilis, and semitendinosus muscles: These are three tendons situated on the posteromedial side of the knee, which insert into the lower portion of the medial tibial plateau. They mainly provide for stability to the medial side of the knee joint during valgus stress. These tendons are like a goat's foot and therefore called pes anserinus. The semitendinosus tendon is the most posterior and inferior of the lot, with the gracilis tendon lying anterior and medial to it. The sartorius muscle is a wide, thick strap-like band just above the gracilis tendon.

At the common insertion of these tendons is seen a bursa which lies beneath it called the pes anserinus bursa, which may be inflamed giving rise to pain. The semitendinosus muscle is sometimes used as a graft to reinforce the medial compartment of the knee joint.

Zone III: Lateral Aspect

Lateral meniscus: This is situated on the lateral aspect of the joint and is less frequently torn as compared with the medial meniscus. The meniscus is attached to the popliteus muscle and not to the lateral collateral ligament, thus making it more mobile than the medial meniscus. The lateral meniscus is a common site for the development of a cyst which can be felt as a firm and tender mass.

Lateral collateral ligament: This is a stout cord which originates from the lateral femoral condyle to be inserted into the head of the fibula. This is palpated easily when the knee is flexed to 90° and the hip is abducted and laterally rotated to relax the iliotibial tract.

Anterior superior tibiofibular ligament: This lies in the interval between the tibia and the fibular head. It is rarely pathologically involved.

Biceps femoris tendon: This is palpated when the knee is flexed at which point it becomes taut and can be felt on the lateral side at its insertion to the fibular head.

Iliotibial tract: This tract is situated just anterior to the lateral aspect of the knee joint and is inserted into the lateral tibial tubercle. This is neither a muscle nor a tendon but a thick band of fascia, and contractures of this can result from paralytic cases like poliomyelitis and meningomyelocele.

Common peroneal nerve: This nerve can be palpated by rolling it beneath the finger as it winds around the neck of the fibula. Excessive pressure on it may cause a foot drop.

Zone IV: Posterior Aspect

The posterior aspect is marked by the popliteal fossa, which is bordered by the biceps tendon on its lateral side. The medial border is formed by the tendons of the semitendinosus and semimembranosus at its superior medial border, while the inferior borders are formed by the origin of the heads of the gastrocnemius muscle. A group of neurovascular structures cross beneath it to the leg.

Posterior tibial nerve: This is a branch of the sciatic nerve and is the most superficial structure in the popliteal fossa.

The popliteal vein: This vein lies directly beneath the nerve.

The popliteal artery: This lies very deep in contact with the joint capsule of the knee joint. Quite commonly seen in the popliteal fossa is the popliteal cyst or Baker's cyst which is a painless mobile swelling seen on the medial side of the fossa and is a distention of the gastrocnemius-semimembranosus bursa.

Gastrocnemius muscle: Both the heads of the muscle are palpable at its origin when the knee is flexed against resistance.

Tests for Joint Stability

Collateral ligaments: These are tested by the patient lying supine with knees extended. The collaterals are tested with the knees in 10° of flexion. The knee to be tested is held with the limb straight, and the other hand placed over the lateral side of the joint over the head of the fibula. This hand is pushed medially while the limb is pulled laterally to create a valgus stress. During this maneuver, the joint space can be palpated for a slight widening. Releasing of that pressure may elicit a clunk which is felt in the tibia and femur closing against each other. This test can be done conversely for a varus stress of the knee, which will demonstrate instability of the lateral side of the knee joint. Since the medial collateral ligament is more important to stability than the lateral one, an isolated tear there may cause joint instability, whereas a similar isolated tear of the lateral collateral ligament may not be enough to cause joint instability. This is the reason most tears occur on the medial side of the knee joint.

Cruciate ligaments: Both these ligaments are very important in preventing anterior and posterior dislocations of the knee joint, and they both are intracapsular originating on the tibia and inserted onto the inner sides of the femoral condyles.

These are tested by the patient lying supine on the bed with feet kept flat and the knees flexed to 90°. The hamstrings are then tested over the posterior aspect of the knee to ensure that they are not taut. The hands are placed on the knee so that the tibia is pulled anteriorly when it may slide forward under the femur giving a positive anterior drawer sign. This indicates a tear of the anterior cruciate ligament. This test is now repeated with the foot held in internal and external rotation to keep the capsule tight. External rotation of the leg holds the posteromedial capsule tight, and the anterior slide is diminished even if the anterior cruciate is torn. If there is an anterior slide demonstrable, which is equal to that seen with the leg in the neutral position, then both the anterior and posterior cruciates are torn, along with the posteromedial capsule. In such cases the medial collateral ligament may also be torn. Similarly internal rotation of the leg tightens the posterolateral capsule, and forward movement of the leg is reduced when compared with the forward movement, which is reduced when the leg is in the neutral position. This indicates that both the cruciates

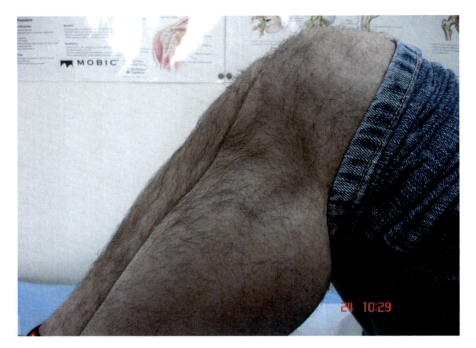

Fig. 6.1 Clinical photograph showing sagging of the tibia posteriorly, indicative of a posterior cruciate tear (Courtesy Dilip Malhotra, Bahrain)

are torn along with the posterolateral capsule of the knee joint. The anterior cruciate ligament may be torn with tears of the medial collateral ligament. Similar tests can be carried out on the posterior cruciate ligament when the tibia is pushed backward to elicit a positive drawer sign in tears of the posterior cruciate ligament (Fig. 6.1). Isolated tears of the posterior cruciate ligament are very rare. The incidence rate of anterior cruciate tears is more than that of posterior cruciate tears.

Range of Motion

There are three basic movements that are seen in the knee joint: namely, flexion, extension, and rotation, including internal and lateral rotations. Flexion and extension are mainly the result of movement between the femur and the tibia. Rotations involve displacement of the menisci on the tibia, along with movement between the tibia and the femur. Extension is performed by the quadriceps, while flexion is performed by the hamstrings along with gravity. Internal and external rotations are done when the knee is slightly flexed by the semimembranosus, semitendinosus, gracilis, and sartorius on the medial side. It is done on the lateral side by the biceps.

Active Range of Movement

Flexion: Ask the patient to squat down on the floor. He should be able to do this with his knees flexed.

Extension: Ask the patient to stand up from the sitting position and he should be able to do this in standing up. Also ask the patient to sit on the table and extend his knee fully. Normally he should be able to extend his knee fully, but in some cases, this movement may not be complete for the last 15°, in which case it is called as an "extensor lag" – something that is commonly seen in quadriceps weakness. It is important to note that some amount of external rotation of the tibia on the femur occurs when the knee is fully extended. This is explained by the anatomic configuration of the knee joint, with the medial femoral condyle being half an inch longer than the lateral femoral condyle. This can be seen in the screw home movement which is seen from a pencil dot over the midpoint of the patella and the tibial tubercle. Now ask the patient to bend and extend the knee joint. The tibial tubercle turns slightly laterally on full extension, and this may be prevented by a torn meniscus.

Internal and external rotations: Ask the patient to rotate his foot medially and laterally, which should be possible to 10° on either side.

Passive Range of Movement

Flexion is possible to 135° when the heel touches the posterior aspect of the thigh. Extension should be full in both the knees to 0°, but occasionally slight hyperextension may be seen. Internal and external rotations are possible to 10° and are tested with both knees held straight with the hands on the ankles rotating the legs.

Neurologic Examination

Muscle Testing

Extension – primary extensor – quadriceps – femoral nerve – L2, L3, L4

Flexion – primary flexor:

1. Semitendinosus-tibial portion of the sciatic nerve – L5
2. Semimembranosus-tibial portion of the sciatic nerve – L5
3. Biceps femoris-tibial portion of the sciatic nerve – S1

These are tested by asking the patient to lie supine on the examining bed and to flex the knee. Then ask the patient to extend her knee with gradually increasing resistance to test the quadriceps muscle. To test the flexors, mainly biceps on the lateral side, externally rotate the leg while flexing the knee against resistance.

Similarly the semitendinosus and semimembranosus on the medial side can be tested with the leg internally rotated. Tests for internal and external rotation are made together with those for flexion and extension.

Sensation Testing

The sensory dermatomes of the knee run in long oblique bands as follows:

1. L4 crosses the anterior aspect of the knee continuing down the medial side of the leg. This is the infrapatellar branch of the saphenous nerve, which supplies the skin over the medial femoral condyle. It is commonly cut during medial meniscectomy.
2. L3 supplies the anterior aspect of the thigh just at and above the knee joint. This is mainly supplied by the femoral nerve.
3. L2 supplies the anterior aspect of the middle of the thigh, by the femoral nerve.
4. S2 supplies a strip of the middle of the posterior thigh and the popliteal fossa by the posterior cutaneous nerve of the thigh.

Reflex Testing

The only reflex to be tested is the patellar reflex – L2, L3, L4

For clinical purposes, the patellar reflex is considered to be an L4 reflex. This reflex is tested by asking the patient to be seated with his legs dangling free on the side or with one leg crossed over the other. When the patient is lying down, the knee joint is held in slight flexion while testing this reflex. The tendon is tapped to elicit the reflex, and reinforcing this may be helpful.

Special Tests

McMurray's test: This is performed for a torn meniscus, and the click may be audible during movements of flexion and extension. Ask the patient to lie down supine on the bed while doing the test. With the leg held with one hand, the knee is flexed to 90°. The leg is then internally and externally rotated initially to loosen the meniscus. Press on the lateral side to apply a valgus strain while externally rotating the leg. Maintaining the valgus strain and external rotation, gradually extend the knee with the finger placed over the medial joint line. This maneuver may cause a palpable or audible click due to a torn meniscus.

Apley's compression or grinding test: Ask the patient to lie prone on the bed and flex her knee to 90°. Now rotate the knee internally and externally while compressing the leg. This will elicit pain which is localized to the medial aspect of the knee to indicate a torn meniscus.

Distraction test: This test mainly differentiates meniscal tears and ligamentous pathology of the knee joint and is done in continuation of the compression test. Applying traction to the leg while rotating it with internal and external rotation will decrease pressure over a torn meniscus and increase pressure over the medial and lateral collateral ligaments, causing pain.

Reduction click: This is a test done to reduce a torn meniscus in a locked knee. This is tested by asking the patient to lie down on the bed and gently rotate the knee internally and externally to help the torn meniscus slip back into place until the knee extends fully with an audible click, thus unlocking the knee joint.

"Bounce home" test: This test is done to demonstrate full extension of the knee in a torn meniscus or with a foreign body in the knee. Ask the patient to flex his knee fully and then passively start to extend the knee slowly. The knee will extend fully or may bounce back into full extension after a sharp end point.

Patella femoral grinding test: This is mainly to determine the integrity of the articulating surfaces of the patella and the articular groove of the distal femur. This is tested by first pushing the patella distally in the groove while asking the patient to tighten her quadriceps. Palpate the movement of the patella which should be smooth and gliding in normal cases. However, if the test is positive, the patient will complains of pain and discomfort, and clinically there will be pain on climbing stairs.

Apprehension test for patellar dislocation and subluxation: This test mainly elicits a feeling of apprehension on the patient's face when the patella is maneuvered to dislocate it laterally.

Tinnel's sign: This can be elicited by tapping or percussing over the cut end of a nerve or provocation of pain on a regenerating nerve. This test is mainly positive around the medial area of the knee where the infrapatellar branch of the saphenous nerve is located and which is invariably cut during medial meniscectomy resulting in a neuroma which is painful.

Tests for Knee Joint Effusion: Tests for major knee joint effusion: Examine the knee joint extended with the patient lying down on the bed and the quadriceps relaxed. Push the patella distally into the trochlear groove which is held there in place by the other hand in the suprapatellar pouch. If the patella is felt to be ballotable, this is an indication of a major knee joint effusion.

Tests for a minor effusion: With the patient lying on the bed with the knee extended, the medial part of the knee joint is milked out to observe filling of the lateral aspect of the knee joint.

Examination of Related Areas

Examination of the lower limb is complete with examination of the joint above and below, which should be complete and thorough for any referred pain at the knee.

Certain specific conditions affecting the knee joint should be kept in mind while examining the knee joint.

Fig. 6.2 Clinical photograph of genu
valgum left knee (Courtesy Dilip
Malhotra, Bahrain)

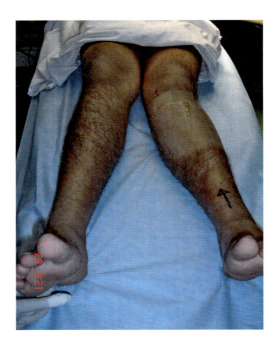

1. Deformities of the knee.

   (a) *Knock knee or genu valgum*: This is the commonest deformity of the knee
       and is usually bilateral and idiopathic, and may be seen in rickets, rheuma-
       toid arthritis, and other neurologic disorders. Radiographs are very helpful in
       this condition (Fig. 6.2), and the child is usually seen at an interval of
       3 months to monitor progress. Raising the inner heel may be helpful in some
       cases to relieve the strain, and stapling the inner side of the knee epiphysis
       may help in arresting the disorder. A low femoral osteotomy may be worth
       considering in cases where a caliper has been tried.

   (b) *Bow legs (genu varum)*: This is usually seen as idiopathic or in rickets and
       certain epiphyseal injuries of the upper tibia (Fig. 6.3). A special variety
       called Blount's disease is seen in the West Indies, when the posteromedial
       aspect of the proximal tibial epiphysis fails to grow normally (Fig. 6.4).
       Clinically the deformity is the only symptom, and radiographs are very useful
       in these cases. Usually these cases recover untreated, but sometimes closed
       osteoclasis of the tibia, stapling the outer side of the lower femoral epiphysis,
       or even an upper tibial osteotomy may be considered in certain cases.

   (c) *Hyperextension of the knee (genu recurvatum)*: This condition may be con-
       genital or may be seen in rickets or in cases of lax ligaments. The condition
       is mainly symptomless, and deformity is the main complaint. Treatment for
       this condition is by means of calipers and treatment of the underlying cause.

Fig. 6.3 Clinical photograph
of bilateral genu varum
(Courtesy Dilip Malhotra,
Bahrain)

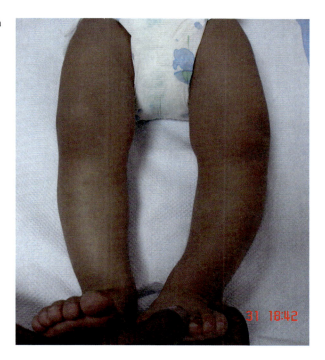

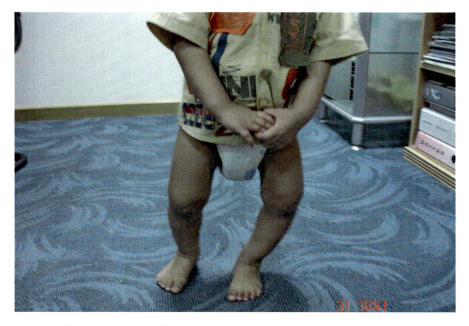

Fig. 6.4 Clinical photograph of Blount's disease in left knee (Courtesy Dilip Malhotra, Bahrain)

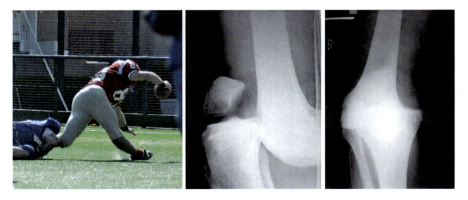

Fig. 6.5 Severe ligamentous injury of the knee with dislocation of the knee (Photograph and X-rays courtesy of M. A. Syed, Kent, UK)

2. Swellings of the knee.

   (a) *Traumatic synovitis*: Here the fluid pushes the patella forward, which is seen very clearly on radiographs, and treatment is usually by quadriceps exercises along with a crepe bandage or back splint if necessary.
   (b) *Nontraumatic synovitis*: Here the synovitis occurs without any injury. This may be seen in acute or chronic cases of inflammation or in transient synovitis.
   (c) *Hemarthrosis*: Without any obvious injury, this represents a case of hemophilia. The knee joint is filled within a matter of hours. Aspiration under sterile conditions will confirm the diagnosis. Quadriceps exercises and a crepe bandage or a back splint may be helpful in certain cases.
   (d) *Tuberculosis of the knee joint*: This is usually the result of a blood-borne infection and starts off as a synovitis which may progress to arthritis with fibrosis. Sinuses are fairly common as the knee joint is superficial. In the early stages, radiographs may show rarefaction. Gradually the joint space decreases when arthritis supervenes. In the early stages of the active disease, traction on a Thomas' splint is very useful. In the healing stages, a weight-relieving caliper or a removable polythene splint is helpful. In the healed stage, a Charnley's arthrodesis using compression clamps is the method of choice.

3. Ligament injuries: Most ligament injuries occur when the knee is bent (Fig. 6.5), and various classifications are given for this injury depending on which quadrant of the knee joint is involved. These injuries may be complete or partial tears and the knee is examined in three main ways: sideways tilting with the knee bent to about 30° of flexion, anteroposterior gliding with the leg rotated medially and laterally, and finally rotation of the flexed knee tested in all directions. All of these movements are then compared with those of the other knee. Radiographs are very useful when the ligament is avulsed with a piece of bone, and stress films are carried out when necessary. Partial tears are treated by aspiration of the hemarthrosis and a plaster cast or a back splint, to permit regular examination at

Fig. 6.6 Arthroscopy showing a torn medial meniscus (Courtesy Dushyant H. Thakkar, London, UK)

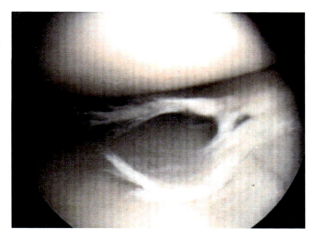

weekly intervals. Complete tears are usually treated by operative intervention. The operative procedure may be carried out in 2 weeks with a generous incision. Repair of every torn structure is carried out, which is finally protected by an above-knee plaster with the knee joint kept in about 30° of flexion. Various surgical operations are known for ligament injuries, and most importantly adhesions and instability are avoided by these procedures.

4. Meniscal injuries

   (a) *Torn medial meniscus*: This is the most commonly torn meniscus, and the tear may be in the anterior horn, posterior horn, or both. This torn part may be displaced inward into the knee joint, resulting in locking of the knee joint when the knee is extended, thereby blocking extension. An accurate history of a twisting force on a bent knee as seen commonly in footballers is of vital importance. Radiographs are normal, but arthrography may reveal the tear (Fig. 6.6). It is very important to differentiate between true locking and pseudo-locking. Treatment is mainly conservative in the first instance by quadriceps exercises and manipulation when the knee is locked. Surgical treatment in the form of excision of the medial meniscus is indicated when the symptoms are recurrent or if the joint cannot be unlocked.

   (b) *Other meniscal lesions*: These lesions must be kept in mind as they are seen less frequently. A torn lateral meniscus is less often seen on account of its greater mobility. An immobile meniscus is seen in the elderly, and a discoid lateral meniscus which is usually recognized by its characteristic loud clunk noise may occasionally be seen. Meniscal cysts are sometimes seen, and they most often occur in the lateral meniscus, where they are treated by an excision of the lateral meniscus.

5. Extensor mechanism lesions:

   (a) Strains, avulsions, and ruptures may be seen in resisted extension of the knee, and this presents in different ways depending on the age of the patient.

Fig. 6.7 Lateral radiograph
of the knee joint showing a
transverse fracture of the
patella (Courtesy Dilip
Malhotra, Bahrain)

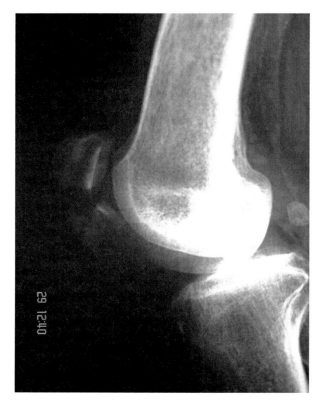

When it is above the patella in the elderly, a transverse fracture of the patella
in the middle-aged is indicated (Fig. 6.7), and a torn patellar ligament in the
younger age groups. Osgood–Schlatter's disease is a commonly seen entity
in children and is a variety of osteochondritis, when a tender bony lump may
be felt over the tibial apophyses, and radiographs show fragmentation of the
apophyses. Spontaneous recovery is often seen by restricting strenuous
activity for a short period of time.

(b) *Recurrent dislocation of the patella*: This is commonly seen in adolescent
children due to lax ligaments, weak muscles, or anatomic abnormalities. The
dislocation is always to the lateral side, and treatment is usually conservative
in the first few instances by rest and quadriceps exercises. Only when the
dislocation is recurrent is an operation considered. Surgical treatment by
lateral release and medial reefing is a soft tissue procedure with excellent
results, and in some cases realignment of the patellar tendon or even a patel-
lectomy can be considered. Recurrent subluxation of the patella is more
common than a recurrent dislocation, and it is treated along similar lines.

(c) *Chondromalacia patellae*: This is commonly seen in young adolescent girls
with tenderness behind the patellae and is usually caused by softening of the

Fig. 6.8 Arthroscopy showing chondromalacia patellae (Courtesy Dushyant H. Thakkar, London, UK)

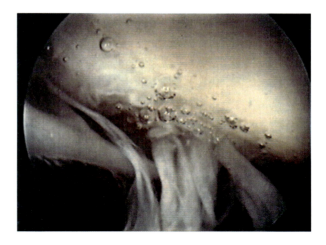

articular cartilage behind the patellae. Skyline radiographs of the knee may be helpful in diagnosing the condition. Treatment is initially conservative by avoiding violent activity, with quadriceps strengthening exercises along with heat in the form of short-wave diathermy. In refractory cases, an operation can be considered (Fig. 6.8).

(d) *Quadriceps contracture*: Here the quadriceps muscle becomes fibrosed and shortened. This may be seen in children following injections into the anterior aspect of the thigh. The vastus intermedius is commonly involved, and treatment is by division of the affected muscle.

6. Other disorders of the knee:

(a) *Bursae*: These are commonly seen in the prepatellar bursa (housemaid's knee) or infrapatellar bursitis (clergyman's knee) or semimembranosus bursa may occur due to constant repetitive friction.

(b) *Loose bodies*: These may occur due to injury, degeneration, or inflammation and may be symptomless in many cases. Treatment by surgical removal is only considered when they cause symptoms such as locking.

(c) *Osteochondritis dissecans*: This is usually caused by trauma when an osteochondral fracture remains ununited (Fig. 6.9). The medial surface of the femoral condyle is a very common site for this to occur and is clearly seen on radiographs. With time, spontaneous healing can occur, but when the healing is uncertain, then surgical drilling of the crater after excision of the loose fragment is advocated.

(d) *Osteoarthritis of the knee*: This is fairly common, with the lower limb having a varus deformity along with pain and tenderness along the medial joint line (Fig. 6.10). Radiographs are very useful in determining the extent of medial compartment narrowing, and conservative treatment is usually not satisfactory. When conservative treatment does fail, surgical treatment in the

Fig. 6.9 Arthroscopy showing an osteochondritis dissecans lesion (Courtesy Dushyant H. Thakkar, London, UK)

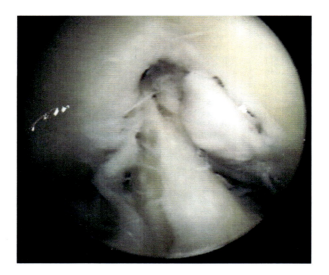

Fig. 6.10 Arthroscopy showing medial compartment osteoarthritis of the knee joint (Courtesy Dushyant H. Thakkar, London, UK)

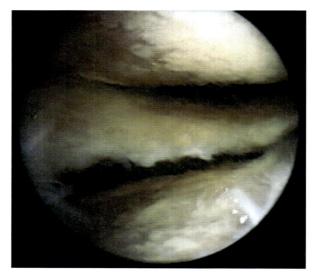

form of an osteotomy, arthrodesis, or arthroplasty can be carried out (Fig. 6.11). In some select cases where the arthritis is mainly confined to the patellofemoral joint, a patellofemoral replacement may be carried out with relief of pain (Fig. 6.12).

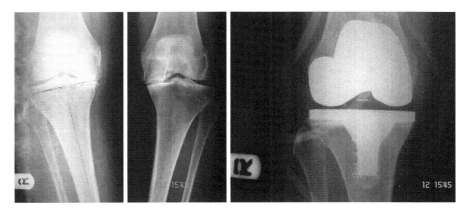

Fig. 6.11 Radiographs of the knee joint showing medial compartment osteoarthritis treated by total knee replacement (Courtesy Dilip Malhotra, Bahrain)

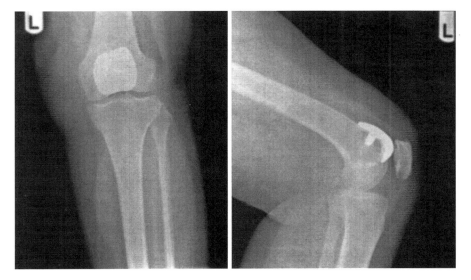

Fig. 6.12 Anteroposterior and lateral radiographs of the knee joint showing patellofemoral replacement (Courtesy Dushyant H. Thakkar, London, UK)

(e) *Charcot's disease*: This is usually caused by repetitive trauma to an insensitive joint, when the joint becomes disorganized and lax with calcified masses in the capsule. Arthrodesis is usually very difficult in these cases, and a caliper is the treatment of choice, because of instability.

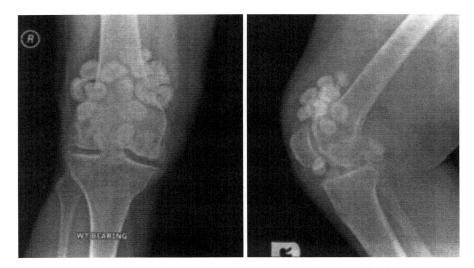

Fig. 6.13 Anteroposterior and lateral radiographs of the right knee showing synovial osteochondromatosis (Courtesy Dushyant H. Thakkar, London, UK)

 (f) *Synovial osteochondromatosis*: This is a condition which is seen in men above the age of 40 years. It usually affects bigger joints such as the knee. It presents as a synovitis, and X-rays taken may show the condition (Fig. 6.13), but when not seen in the early stages, magnetic resonance imaging is useful for its diagnosis.

Chapter 7
Examination of the Foot and Ankle

Inspection

This is done from the moment a patient enters the examining room. A deformed foot may be seen in a deformed shoe when the patient walks into the examining room. Certain examples are as follows: The shoes of a patient with drop foot show scuffed toes due to scrapping the floor in the swing phase. Similarly a patient with a toe-in shows excessive wear over the lateral border of the sole. Inspection is started in the normal manner with the counting of the toes, as in some cases an extra toe may be seen (supernumerary toe or digit). A disproportionately large great toe may be seen which is swollen or as a congenital anomaly.

The normal foot when seen at rest has some degree of plantarflexion and inversion as opposed to spastic feet which show dorsiflexion and eversion. The normal foot has a dome due to the medial longitudinal arch, which extends between the first metatarsal and the calcaneus. This arch is abnormally high in pes cavus or may be absent in pes planus. Occasionally in children, the forefoot is seen to be deviated medially on the hindfoot to cause a forefoot adductus deformity.

Observe if there are any changes in the color of the foot in weight-bearing and non-weight-bearing positions. Diagnosis of arterial insufficiency may be thought of when the foot which was light pink when elevated is beet red on being lowered (dependent rubor).

The skin of the foot is normally thick in weight-bearing areas such as the base of the first metatarsal head or the calcaneus. This may be increased in pathologic conditions, when it is called a callosity as is seen in weight-bearing regions of the foot. The foot and the ankle are also examined for either a unilateral or bilateral swelling. This may be seen in trauma, or cases of bilateral swelling may be seen in lymphatic obstruction in cardiac or pelvic pathology. This is normally seen just above the medial malleolus as a pitting edema.

K M. Iyer, *Clinical Examination in Orthopedics*,
DOI 10.1007/978-0-85729-971-0_7, © Springer-Verlag London Limited 2012

Palpation: Bony Points

1. *Medial aspect*: The head of the first metatarsal and the first metatarsophalangeal joint are palpable as the ball of the foot. Occasionally bony prominences may be palpated over the metatarsal head in certain conditions such as gout and bunions. The first metatarsal bone extends proximally as a flare at its base until the first metatarsocuneiform bone.

   Continuing proximally is the navicular bone which articulates distally with the three cuneiform bones, laterally with the cuboid bone, and proximally with the talus. Occasionally aseptic necrosis of the navicular may be seen as a tender area in children, and in some, an additional bone which is prominent and tender may be felt attached to the navicular. This is known as the accessory navicular bone. The head of the talus lies just proximal to the navicular, which becomes more prominent on eversion of the ankle.

   Continuing with palpation over the medial side, the medial malleolus is felt as a prominence which articulates with one-third of the medial side of the talus. Continuing plantarward is the sustentaculum tali which is a bony prominence providing attachment to the spring ligament and which may cause pes planus if deficient. The medial tubercle of the talus is a small bony prominence situated immediately posteriorly to the medial malleolus and serves as a point of insertion for the medial collateral ligament of the ankle.

2. *Lateral aspect*: The fifth metatarsal bone and the metatarsal joint are situated on the lateral side of the ball of the foot. The proximal part of the bone ends in a flare called the styloid process into which is inserted the tendon of the peroneus brevis. Just behind the styloid process is a groove on the cuboid in which the tendon of the peroneus longus runs to the medial plantar aspect of the foot. The calcaneus can be easily palpated subcutaneously just proximal along the lateral border of the foot.

   The peroneal tubercle is a bony prominence on the lateral surface of the calcaneus and lies just distal to the lateral malleolus. It separates the tendons of the peroneus brevis and peroneus longus as they pass around the lateral surface of calcaneus. The lateral malleolus which is the distal end of the fibula is situated slightly distally and posteriorly compared with the medial malleolus. It contributes with the medial malleolus to form the ankle mortise which points 15° laterally and is commonly involved in fractures.

Sinus Tarsi Area

This is a depression which lies just anterior to the lateral malleolus and is filled with the extensor digitorum brevis and a pad of fat.

The dome of the talus is palpated with the foot in plantarflexion and inversion. A greater part of this dome is felt on the lateral side as compared with the medial side. Very rarely a defect may be palpable, as in osteochondritis desiccans. The inferior tibiofibular joint is located just proximal to the talus with the anterior tibiofibular ligament overlying this joint.

Area of the Hindfoot

The bare part of the dome of the talus protrudes posteriorly from behind the ankle joint. The medial tubercle of the calcaneus which lies on the medial plantar surface of the calcaneus and is large and broad gives attachment to the abductor hallucis longus muscle medially and to the flexor digitorum brevis and the plantar aponeurosis anteriorly. It may occasionally be seen as a bony spur which is tender on palpation. The medial tubercle of the calcaneum is weight bearing while the lateral tubercle is not. In children the posterior aspect of the calcaneus is tender, which is known as Sever's epiphysitis.

Plantar Surface

This is examined with the plantar surface of the foot facing the examiner. This surface is difficult to examine because of the fascial bands from the palmar aponeurosis which limit palpation of the bony prominences. Palpating from the calcaneus distally along the medial longitudinal arch of the foot toward the great toe, beneath the first metatarsal head is the flexor hallucis brevis tendon which has two sesamoid bones which may be inflamed in some cases giving rise to a sesamoiditis which is tender. Continuing palpation just lateral to the first metatarsal head, the transverse arch of the foot lies and is felt from the first to the fifth metatarsal heads. Occasionally tenderness may be felt over the second metatarsal head in fractures which are quite common in the second metatarsal neck. Occasionally a callosity may be palpated over the fifth metatarsal head.

Soft tissue palpation: This is carried out in various zones:

Zone I: Head of First Metatarsal Bone

This area is the site of a common deformity namely the hallux valgus and bunion. It is a deformity characterized by lateral deviation of the big toe, which in some cases may be so excessive that the big toe may overlap the second toe. In some cases, the first metatarsal may be deviated medially, in a condition called metatarsus primus varus. This may also form a projection of bone over the medial area of the first metatarsal head, and constant friction over this area may result in development of a bursa. This is called a bunion and is tender and inflamed. Sometimes gouty crystals may be deposited in the tissues about the joint, which can cause pain and deformity.

Zone II: Navicular Tubercle and Talar Head

As described previously, the plantar portion of the talar head articulates with the sustentaculum tali and the anterior part of the posterior aspect of the navicular. The talar head which lacks support between these two articulations is supported by the tibialis posterior tendon and the spring ligament which extends from the sustentaculum tali to the navicular. This is clearly seen in pes planus when this support is lost and the talar head displaces medially and plantarward stretching the spring ligament and the tibialis posterior to result in a loss of the longitudinal arch. This is clearly seen as a callosity which develops over the prominent talar head, and results in a valgus angle of the calcaneus especially when viewed from the posterior aspect of the foot.

Zone III: Medial Malleolus

The deltoid ligament is a broad and strong ligament which lies on the medial side of the medial malleolus. Below the deltoid ligament is the medial collateral ligament of the ankle joint. In the depression between the posterior aspect of the medial malleolus and the tendoachilles are the following structures from anterior to posterior: tibialis posterior tendon, flexor digitorum longus tendon, posterior tibial artery and tibial nerve, and flexor hallucis longus tendon.

The tibialis posterior tendon is very prominent when the patient inverts and plantarflexes the foot, when it is visible as it passes behind and inferior to the medial malleolus. In cases of spasticity in poliomyelitis or meningomyelocele in which the other muscles around the ankle are weak, the tibialis posterior stands out as a strong chord causing a plantarflexion and inversion deformity of the foot. The flexor digitorum longus tendon lies just behind the tibialis posterior tendon which can seen when the toes are flexed. The flexor hallucis longus tendon lies on the posterior aspect of the ankle joint where it forms a groove on the posterior aspect of the talus between the medial and lateral tubercles as it crosses the ankle joint. All of these tendons pass very close to each other and are protected by a synovial lining which causes pain when inflamed behind the medial malleolus.

The posterior tibial artery normally runs between the tendons of the flexor digitorum longus and the flexor hallucis longus and is of clinical importance as it is the main blood supply to the foot.

The tibial nerve runs just immediately posterior and lateral to the posterior tibial artery and is of clinical importance as it is the main nerve to the sole of the foot. The nerve and the artery are held to the tibia to form the tarsal tunnel which can be compressed to create neurovascular problems in the foot. The long saphenous vein is seen visibly anterior to the medial malleolus. This may be used for an intravenous infusion when the veins in the upper limb are inaccessible.

Zone IV: Dorsum of the Foot Between the Malleoli

The important structures passing from the medial to the lateral side are as follows: the tibialis posterior tendon, the extensor hallucis longus tendon, dorsalis pedis artery, and extensor digitorum longus tendon. The tibialis anterior tendon is the most medial structure and also the strongest dorsiflexor and invertor of the foot. Weakness in it causes a foot drop. This can be tested easily by asking the patient to dorsiflex his foot when it becomes prominent as it inserts to the medial aspect of the base of the first metatarsal and the first cuneiform bone. The extensor hallucis longus tendon lies just lateral to the tibialis anterior tendon and is palpated by asking the patient to dorsiflex her great toe. This tendon is very useful in tendon transfers for a foot drop, when it is transferred to the dorsum of the foot. The extensor digitorum longus tendon lies just lateral to the extensor hallucis longus as it lies at the ankle joint. Distally it splits into four slips each of which inserts into the dorsal part of the base of the distal phalanx of the toes. These tendons can be palpated when the toes are extended.

The dorsalis pedis artery: This artery lies between the extensor hallucis longus and the extensor digitorum longus tendons as it passes to supply the foot. This artery may be affected in vascular disease.

The tibialis anterior, extensor hallucis longus, and extensor digitorum longus originate from the anterior compartment of the leg between the tibia and the fibula. This anterior compartment is enveloped by a strong anterior fascia covering the posterior tibia, the fibula, and the interosseous membrane, thus rendering it rigid in nature. Sometimes in fractures of the tibia and fibula, a hematoma within the muscles may collect which causes pain within the anterior compartment of the leg causing necrosis of the muscles, nerves, and vessels and resulting in a foot drop. This is also _____ ~artment syndrome.

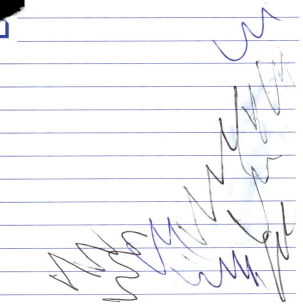

teral side and is not as strong as the medial
parts: The anterior talofibular ligament is
d in an inversion sprain of the ankle joint.
neofibular ligament which is inserted into
is involved only after the first part is also
cted it may lead to ankle instability. The
ent which is inserted into the small poste-
very strong and prevents forward slippage
ed in severe injuries of the ankle.
These two tendons pass over the lateral
ubercle in between them. They are strong
red by a retinaculum which keeps them in
ndons when this retinaculum is deficient.

This may result in snapping tendons when the snap is seen and felt audibly. The peroneus brevis tendon passes below the tubercle and is inserted into the tuberosity of the base of the fifth metatarsal, which may be pulled along with a flake of bone or may fracture when it is tender.

Zone VI: Sinus Tarsi

The sinus tarsi is commonly affected in ankle sprains, rheumatoid arthritis, or spastic paralysis. The extensor digitorum brevis tendon may be felt bulging out of the sinus tarsi when the patient extends his toes.

Zone VII: Head of the Fifth Metatarsal

A bursa is present just overlying the lateral side of the fifth metatarsal. This may be inflamed giving rise to a callosity called a "tailor's bunion."

Zone VIII: Calcaneus

The gastrocnemius and the soleus muscles form a common tendon called the tendoachilles, which is the strongest tendon in the body. This can be ruptured by a sharp blow or a laceration, which is painful and tender and in which case, the patient is unable to perform plantarflexion. The ruptured ends may retract leaving a palpable defect just above the posterior calcaneus. The tendon is tested by asking the patient to lie prone. The calf is squeezed to see if there is any plantarflexion. If it is diminished or absent, the tendon is ruptured.

The retrocalcaneal bursa lies between the tendoachilles and the posterior superior angle of the calcaneus. This can be inflamed in bursitis due to excessive friction over the bursa, such as with ill-fitting shoes.

Calcaneal bursa: This is located superficially between the tendoachilles and the skin of the heel. This can be located by pinching the bursa between the examining fingers.

Zone IX: Plantar Surface of the Foot

The central bony prominence that is felt in the hindfoot is the medial tubercle of the calcaneus. Most of the muscles of the foot originate from it, and it should be examined for the presence of a bony prominence called a calcaneal spur, which is tender on palpation.

Plantar aponeurosis (*plantar fascia*): These are strong bands of fascia which originate at the medial tubercle of the calcaneus splaying out into the sole to be attached to the ligamentous structures near the metatarsal heads in the forefoot. The sole of the foot is normally smooth to palpation but may be nodular in plantar fascitis, when it is painful. Continued palpation between the metatarsal heads for nodules or tenderness. An area of tenderness between the heads of the third and fourth metatarsals is commonly seen. It is called a Morton's neuroma.

Zone X: Toes

Certain pathological conditions which are commonly seen in the toes:

Claw toes: This is a condition which is commonly seen in pes cavus when the metatarsophalangeal joint is hyperextended along with hyperflexion of the proximal and distal interphalangeal joints. In this condition, callosities may develop over the dorsum of the toes and over the metatarsal heads on the plantar side.

Hammer toes: This is usually seen in the second toe and consists of hyperextension of the metatarsophalangeal and distal interphalangeal joints along with hyperflexion of the proximal interphalangeal joint. This is usually seen in patients with ill-fitting shoes.

Corns: Soft corns are usually found due to the excessive moisture between the toes, especially between the fourth and fifth toes. Hard corns are usually felt on the dorsum of the flexed interphalangeal joint, usually the fifth toe.

Ingrown toenails: The anterior corners of the lateral and medial sides of the toenail may dig into the surrounding skin resulting in pain, redness, and tenderness of the soft tissue.

Tests for Ankle Stability

Stability of the ankle joint depends on the integrity of structures on the medial and lateral sides. The most common stress affecting the ankle joint is an inversion stress because of two reasons: (1) the medial malleolus is shorter than the lateral malleolus, thus permitting the talus to invert farther than it can evert, and (2) the ligamentous structures on the lateral side are three separate structures as compared with the deltoid ligament on the medial side (Fig. 7.1).

Both the anterior and posterior stability are tested by the drawer's sign, making the patient sit down with his legs dangling down the edge of the table. One hand is placed over the distal tibia firmly, and the other hand is placed over the calcaneus. The distal tibia is pushed posteriorly while the calcaneus is pulled anteriorly to elicit the anterior drawer sign. Normally the anterior talofibular is tight in all positions, and the anterior drawer sign should be positive if there is anterior forward movement of the talus on the tibia. Conversely, the ankle is tested for posterior stability.

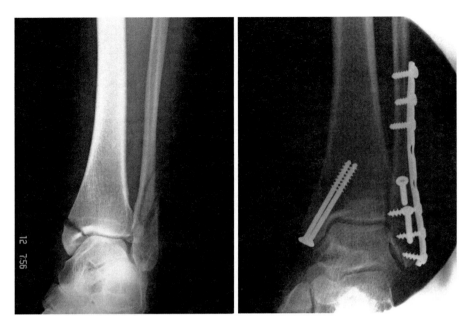

Fig. 7.1 Radiographs of the ankle joint showing a bimalleolar fracture which has been treated by open reduction and internal fixation to restore the congruity of the ankle joint (Courtesy Dilip Malhotra, Bahrain)

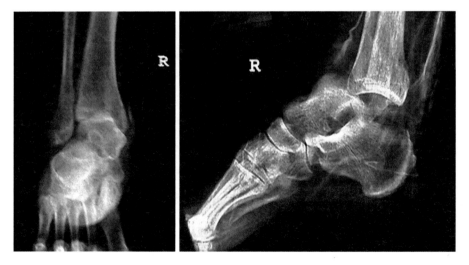

Fig. 7.2 Radiographs showing complete dislocation of the ankle (Courtesy M. A. Syed, Kent, UK)

Both the anterior talofibular and calcaneofibular ligaments must be torn to give rise to gross ankle instability. This is tested by inverting the calcaneus, and if the talus rocks in the ankle mortise, then both these ligaments are torn. The deltoid ligament is tested by everting the calcaneus, with the patient's distal tibia and calcaneus stabilized, when a gap may be felt in the ankle mortise (Fig. 7.2). After completing these clinical tests for ankle stability, a stress X-ray of both sides is taken to confirm the results and to complete the examination.

Range of Motion

The normal range of movements at the foot and ankle are:

1. *Ankle movements*: plantar flexion and dorsiflexion.
2. *Subtalar movements*: inversion and eversion.
3. *Midtarsal movements*: forefoot adduction and forefoot abduction.
4. *Toe movements*: flexion/extension.

Active Range of Movements

Ask the patient to walk on his toes to test for dorsiflexion and ask him to plantarflex his foot and move his toes.

Test for inversion by asking him to walk on the outer border of his foot, and to test for eversion ask him to walk on the inner border of his foot. These are quick active tests in the foot and ankle and inability to perform any of these should make one test the passive range of movements.

Passive Range of Movements

Ankle: Dorsiflexion – 20° and plantarflexion – 50°.

This is tested with the patient sitting at the edge of the table with the knees flexed so that the gastrocnemius is relaxed. Then the movements are tested between the talus and the tibia and fibula. To perform this, first lock the subtalar joint onto the hindfoot in inversion and then plantarflex and dorsiflex the foot to get an idea whether this movement is occurring at the ankle joint only. Decrease in the range of ankle movements may be seen in an extra-articular swelling such as edema following trauma or due to cardiac failure. An intra-articular swelling can also cause restriction of ankle movements such as fusion of the ankle joint or an ankle joint capsular contracture.

Subtalar joint – inversion – 5° and eversion – 5°.

This is tested by holding the distal tibia with the patient sitting on the edge of the table and the calcaneus is held with the other hand and inverted and everted by holding the heel.

Forefoot adduction – 20° and abduction – 10°.

This is tested at the midtarsal joints – namely, the talonavicular joint and the calcaneocuboid joints. This is done by holding the calcaneus with one hand while the other moves the forefoot medially and laterally. Normally these movements are tested independently, though they can be tested in conjunction with inversion and eversion. When forefoot adduction is tested with inversion of the ankle, it is called supination, and when eversion is tested with forefoot abduction, it is called pronation.

First metatarsophalangeal joint – flexion – 45° and extension – 80°.

This joint is extremely important in ambulation in the toe-off phase of gait. This movement may be markedly restricted in certain conditions such as a hallux rigidus or when the joint is fused.

Movements of the lesser toes

Claw toes may cause restriction of extension in the proximal and distal interphalangeal joints and flexion at the metatarsophalangeal joints, while hammer toes cause restriction of flexion in the distal interphalangeal joint, extension at the proximal interphalangeal joint and flexion at the metatarsophalangeal joint.

Neurologic Examination

Muscle Testing

Dorsiflexors:

- Tibialis anterior – deep peroneal nerve – L4 (L5)
- Extensor hallucis longus – deep peroneal nerve – L5
- Extensor digitorum longus – deep peroneal nerve – L5

Tibialis anterior: This is tested by the patient sitting over the edge of the table. The patient tries to force his foot into plantarflexion and eversion with resistance is offered against the first metatarsal and shaft, during which, the muscle is palpated.

Extensor hallucis longus: This is tested by resistance offered in extension of the interphalangeal joint of the great toe over the distal part of the interphalangeal joint. If the finger is placed across the interphalangeal joint, then the extensor hallucis brevis is also tested.

Extensor digitorum longus: This is tested by asking the patient to sit over the edge of the table. The calcaneus is stabilized with one hand, and the other hand tests for extension of the toes against gradually increasing resistance.

Extension digitorum brevis: This muscle is tested as before along with the extensor digitorum longus. Its muscle belly can be palpated in the sinus tarsi where it bulges out.

Plantar Flexors:

1. Peroneus Longus and brevis – superficial peroneal nerve – S1
2. Gastrocnemius and soleus – tibial nerve – S1, S2
3. Flexor hallucis longus – tibial nerve – L5
4. Flexor digitorum longus – tibial nerve – L5
5. Tibialis posterior – tibial nerve – L5

Peroneus longus and brevis: Ask the patient to walk on the medial borders of her feet. This tests the function of both muscles simultaneously, since they are evertors of the foot and the ankle. Passively they are tested by opposing plantar flexion and eversion, gradually increasing resistance against the fifth metatarsal head and shaft.

Gastrocnemius and soleus: The common tendon is tested by asking the patient to walk on his toes.

Flexor hallucis longus: To actively test this muscle, observe the patient's gait. This muscle functions in a smooth toe-off. Alternately, ask the patient to sit at the edge of the table, then ask her to bend or curl her great toe, while opposing this action with a gradually increasing resistance.

Flexor digitorum longus: This test is carried out as above by asking the patient to bend or curl her toes.

Tibialis posterior: This is tested by asking the patient to plantar flex and invert, when he is sitting at the edge of the table. This motion is resisted when the tibialis posterior being stronger can deform the foot.

Sensation Testing:

The L4 dermatome, crossing the knee joint, supplies the medial side of the leg to cover the skin medial to the crest of the tibia, medial malleolus, and medial side of the foot. The L5 dermatome covers the lateral side of the leg lateral to the crest of the tibia and the dorsum of the foot. The S1 dermatome covers the lateral border of the foot.

Reflex Tests: The main reflex to be tested is the Achilles tendon reflex.

Achilles tendon reflex: This is supplied by S1, which is a deep tendon reflex and is mediated through the gastrocnemius muscles. This is tested by reinforcing the reflex, asking the patient to clasp his hands while the test is carried out. If the patient is bedridden, then ask the patient to keep the leg on the opposite leg with the knee hanging. The tendon is put on stretch by dorsiflexion of the foot while the tendon is tapped at the ankle, which elicits the reflex. When the patient is lying prone in bed, flex the knee to 90° and dorsiflex the foot while testing the reflex. If the ankle is swollen or too painful to test this reflex by tapping it, the patient can be asked to lie prone. The ball of the foot is held dorsiflexing the foot, and the reflex can be tested by striking the hammer on the fingers of the hand.

Special Tests

Test for rigid or supple flat feet: This test is observed when the patient stands up on her toes, and while she is seated. If the medial longitudinal arch is absent in all positions, then the patient has rigid flat feet. If on the contrary, the medial longitudinal arch is absent only when the patient stands up, but is present when she is sitting, then the patient has supple flat feet, which are correctible with longitudinal arch supports.

Tibial torsion test: This is commonly seen in children and is diagnosed by an in-toeing gait. Normally a line drawn between the malleoli is externally rotated by 15° to the perpendicular line drawn from the tibial tuberosity to the ankle joint. If internal tibial torsion is excessive and present, then the malleolar line may face anteriorly very close to the perpendicular line.

Forefoot adduction correction test: This test is very useful in children in helping to decide on the future line of treatment by cast correction. If this can be manually corrected beyond the neutral position, then no treatment is necessary for this condition. But if the forefoot can be only partially corrected to the neutral position, then cast correction is needed, as this forefoot will not be corrected without any treatment.

Ankle dorsiflexion test: This is tested by first flexing the knee joint. If it is possible to dorsiflex the ankle, then the gastrocnemius is the muscle causing the limitation since the gastrocnemius is a two-joint muscle which is slackened by relaxation. Because the soleus is a single-joint muscle, flexion of the knee joint will not interfere with dorsiflexion of the ankle joint.

Homan's sign: This test is a valuable indicator for deep vein thrombosis, when forcible dorsiflexion of the ankle elicits pain in the calf muscles. This can be further confirmed by deep palpation of the calf muscle.

Examination of Related Areas

Pain may be referred to the ankle and foot from a pathology of various other joints in the lower limb.

Certain specific conditions must be kept in mind when examining the foot and ankle:

1. *Talipes equinovarus (club foot)*: Here deformity is the only symptom. Genetic and environmental factors are involved, where the talus points downward, the calcaneus faces inward, and the forefoot is adducted. Boys are more often affected than the girls. It is bilateral in one-third of cases and many have other associated congenital deformities (Fig. 7.3). Treatment is usually conservative in the form of stretching and strapping which are started shortly after birth. Resistant cases are operated upon as early as 3–6 weeks after birth. Through a medial incision, the tendoachilles is elongated, along with soft tissue release of the structures

Fig. 7.3 Clinical
photograph showing
bilateral club feet
(Courtesy Dilip Malhotra,
Bahrain)

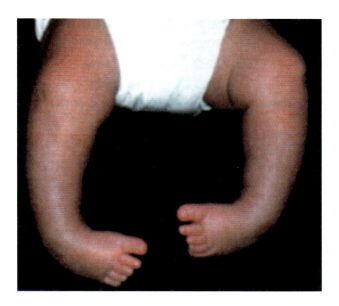

(notably the tight tibialis posterior) on the medial side. After the age of 5 years, a calcaneal Dwyer's osteotomy is very useful, and after age 10, a wedge tarsectomy is the best possible option. Various other deformities of the talipes, such as talipes calcaneus, should be kept in mind when the foot is dorsiflexed with an associated valgus deformity.

2. *The heel*: Two commonly seen conditions must be kept in mind:

   (a) *Ruptured tendoachilles*: This results in a degenerate tendon, when the calf muscle contracts suddenly during running or jumping and is resisted by the body weight. A distinct palpable gap is felt about 4 in. above the ankle, with weak plantarflexion of the ankle joint. The Simmonds' test is also helpful. Complete tears are best treated by operative repair of the tendon.

   (b) *Painful heel*: This condition when seen in children about 10 years of age is known as Sever's disease, which is a mild traction injury. Treatment is by rest and a small heel raise for a few weeks. This condition may also be seen in adolescents and young adults, when it is a bursitis just above the insertion of the tendoachilles. In older adults, this condition is known as a "policeman's heel," and a bony spur may be seen on radiographs. It usually settles down with an injection of hydrocortisone.

3. *The arch*:

   (a) The body weight is transmitted through two columns, with the medial border raised above the ground as an arch of a bridge. Flat foot merely implies that this arch has collapsed inward, as seen in many conditions such as (1) anatomic conditions such as rotation of the limbs, genu valgum, equinus deformity, varus deformity, or congenital. It may also be seen in (2) physiologic conditions such as infantile flat foot, postural flat foot, middle-aged flat foot, and temporary flat foot. There are no symptoms, and this condition is usually spotted by the school doctor or the mother of the affected child. The foot is examined in great detail, and usually treatment is by exercises and arch supports.

(b) *Spasmodic flat foot*: Here the foot is everted, and the muscles are in spasm. Very rarely there may be an abnormal bar of bone which may be demonstrated on special X-ray views. Here, pain is the presenting symptom, and initial conservative treatment is by a below-knee walking plaster cast with the foot in the normal position for 6 weeks. Occasionally a calcaneal bar may be excised in some cases.

(c) *Painful tarsus*: In children, the navicular may becomes dense and fragmented, to give a painful limp. Treatment of this condition is by strapping the foot, along with restricting activity. Eventually the foot becomes completely normal clinically and radiologically, with disappearance of symptoms.

(d) *Pes cavus*: This is usually seen when there is muscular imbalance due to a neurologic disorder or myopathy. This deformity is usually first seen by the mother or the school doctor, with painful callosities, and both feet are affected. Usually this condition is idiopathic but care should be taken to differentiate it from neurologic disorders, myopathies, and Volkmann's ischemia. Treatment of this condition is usually by strengthening the intrinsic muscles with exercises, and in older children, a calcaneal osteotomy combined with release of the plantar fascia and special padded shoes may be helpful.

4. *The hallux*:

(a) *Hallux valgus*: This deformity is usually bilateral and found mostly in females. The basic deformity is a varus of the first metatarsal with an increased width of the forefoot, along with an inflamed bunion at the metatarsophalangeal (MTP) joint (Fig. 7.4). Various forms of treatment are available, since deformity is the only symptom, an alteration in footwear is always considered before surgery, which takes the form of an arthroplasty, of which Keller's operation is the most common and most popular procedure. Various other procedures may be helpful such as a bunionectomy, an osteotomy of the first metatarsal or an arthrodesis of the MTP joint.

(b) *Hallux rigidus*: This condition is usually bilateral with a straight long hallux and a knobbly MTP joint the movements of which are restricted (Fig. 7.5). Treatment is usually by alteration of the footwear and a metatarsal bar, before considering surgery in the form of a Keller's procedure or an arthrodesis of the MTP joint.

(c) *Other disorders of the hallux*: Certain other disorders of the hallux such as gout, seasamoid chondromalacia, or certain toenail disorders such as an ingrown toenail or an overgrown toenail must be kept in mind when examining the hallux.

Fig. 7.4 Clinical photograph showing hallux valgus with a bunion (Courtesy Dilip Malhotra, Bahrain)

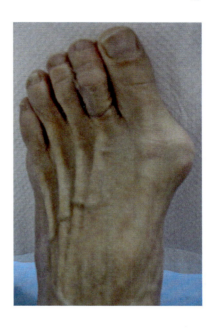

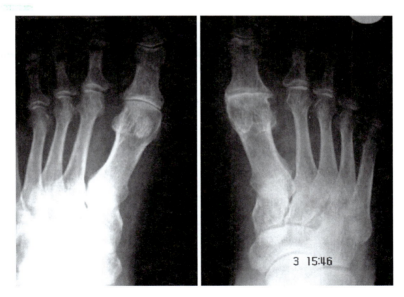

Fig. 7.5 Anteroposterior radiograph of both feet, showing hallux rigidus of the right great toe (Courtesy Dilip Malhotra, Bahrain)

Fig. 7.6 Clinical
photograph showing
hammer toes. The arrow in
the photograph indicates the
side to be operated (*Right
side*) (Courtesy
Dilip Malhotra, Bahrain)

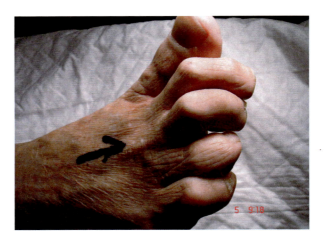

5. *The metatarsal and toes*:

   (a) *Metatarsalgia*: This is a very vague term and includes many varieties such as
       (i) Freiberg's disease, which is a crushing type of osteochondritis of the sec-
       ond metatarsal head, easily diagnosed on radiographs; (ii) stress fracture
       which is usually seen in the neck of the second metatarsal and for which
       radiographs are very helpful in diagnosis; (iii) Morton's metatarsalgia, which
       usually develops in a neuroma of the digital nerve at the level of the metatar-
       sal heads. All of these conditions give rise to metatarsalgia, and treatment is
       mainly by alteration of the footwear along with exercises. Treatment is
       mainly directed toward the cause, such as excision of the Morton's metatar-
       salgia through a plantar incision.
   (b) *Toe disorders*: Affections of the toes may result in hammer toes (Fig. 7.6),
       curly toes or overlapping fifth toes, all of which must be kept in mind.

Chapter 8
Examination of the Cervical Spine

Examination of the cervical spine is done by inspection, palpation, neurologic examination, and certain special tests which are very helpful. The cervical spine has three main functions: Firstly it provides support to stabilize the head, secondly it allows for a range of movements of the head and thirdly it helps to lodge the spinal cord and the vertebral artery.

Inspection and Palpation

The cervical spine is inspected both anteriorly and posteriorly. Anteriorly the salient points are the following:

1. *The hyoid bone*: This is a horseshoe-shaped bony landmark which is situated just above the thyroid cartilage and is at the level of the C3 vertebral body anteriorly. It has two long, thin processes laterally which start in the midline anteriorly and proceed posterolaterally. The bone can be palpated best by placing the examining hand on it while asking the patient to swallow .
2. *Thyroid cartilage*: Proceeding inferiorly, this structure can be palpated to the level of the C4 vertebral body. The anterior portion in its upper part is commonly called the Adam's apple.
3. *The first cricoid ring and the carotid tubercle*: Proceeding slightly inferiorly is the first cricoid ring which lies opposite the C6 vertebral body. It is the only complete ring which is a part of the trachea and just above is the site for an emergency tracheostomy. Too much pressure in palpating this bony landmark may cause gagging of the patient, and it is possible to palpate it, though with less obvious effect than with the thyroid cartilage, by asking the patient to swallow. Proceeding slightly laterally at the level of the cricoid cartilage is the carotid tubercle, which is the anterior tubercle of the transverse process of C6. This forms an anatomic landmark for the anterior surgical approach to the C5-C6 and a mark for the injection of the stellate cervical ganglion.

K M. Iyer, *Clinical Examination in Orthopedics*,
DOI 10.1007/978-0-85729-971-0_8, © Springer-Verlag London Limited 2012

The soft tissues that can be seen and palpated in the anterior aspect are as follows:

1. *Sternocleidomastoid muscle*: This muscle extends from the sternoclavicular joint to the mastoid process and can be palpated by asking the patient to turn the head to the opposite side so that the muscle is taut at its tendinous margin.
2. *Lymph node chain*: These lymph nodes are usually located near the medial border of the sternocleidomastoid and are usually not felt when they are normal. They are only felt when they are enlarged and painful, which indicates some infection in the upper respiratory tract and may even cause torticollis.
3. *Thyroid gland*: This is situated just above the thyroid cartilage in the midline in an H-shaped fashion, with two lobes situated laterally and a thin isthmus connecting them. When enlarged, they may be felt as cysts or nodules which are tender on palpation.
4. *Carotid pulse*: This can be felt over the carotid artery which lies just next to the carotid tubercle. Palpate one artery at a time, for simultaneous palpation of both may induce carotid reflux.
5. *Parotid gland*: This covers the sharp inferior angle of the mandible. Usually it is not palpated distinctly, but when enlarged it may be felt as a boggy swelling (e.g., in mumps) which is not defined and sharp.
6. *Supraclavicular fossa*: This is located just above the mid clavicle and to the lateral aspect of the suprasternal notch. It is covered by the platysma and normally is seen as a smooth indentation. Enlarged glands may be palpated in the fossa, or the smooth indentation may be lost in cases of surgical emphysema where a surgical crepitus may be elicited. A cervical rib when present in the supraclavicular fossa may cause neurologic symptoms in the upper limb.

The posterior aspect of the cervical spine is best examined by one standing behind the patient with the thumbs of the hands on the midline. The structures seen and felt from above downward are:

1. *Occiput*: This is seen and felt with ease.
2. *Inion*: This is a dome-shaped bump which is in the occipital region, and it corresponds to the center of the superior nuchal line.
3. *Superior nuchal line*: This is a transverse ridge which can be felt extending on the lateral sides of the inion on deep palpation.
4. *Mastoid process*: This is a small rounded process felt at the lateral edge of the superior nuchal line.
5. *The spinous processes of the cervical vertebrae*: These are felt in the midline from the base of the occiput downward. These take the shape of a normal lordosis, and the first spinous process is identified as bifid in nature. These bifid spinous processes may be felt in the lower part of the cervical spine as lateral soft tissue bulges, where they are less prominent in nature.
6. *Facet joints*: These are clearly felt about an inch lateral to the midline on both sides. They may not be clearly felt until the patient is relaxed completely. They can then be felt from below the occiput to C7-T1.

The soft tissues that can be palpated in the posterior aspect are as follows:

1. *Trapezius muscle*: This is a broad muscle which originates from the inion and extends to the spine of T12 and laterally to be inserted in an arc to the clavicle, acromion, and the spine of the scapula. This muscle is best palpated bilaterally, as it helps to compare the two sides. Embryologically the trapezius and the sternocleidomastoid form one muscle but split during later development into two muscles. On account of their common origin, they share the same nerve supply from the cranial nerve IX.
2. *Lymph nodes*: These are not usually seen or felt, but when they occur may make one suspicious of infection or tuberculosis.
3. *Greater occipital nerves*: These are felt only when inflamed, just lateral to the inion, which normally results in headache.
4. *Superior nuchal ligament*: This extends from the base of the skull along the spinous processes till the spinal process of C7.

Range of Movements

The range of movements possible in the cervical spine are flexion, extension, lateral rotations, and lateral bending.

About 50% of the lateral rotational movement occurs at C12, between the atlas and the axis, while the rest is evenly distributed among the remaining five cervical vertebrae. This is possible because of the specialized shape of the atlas and axis to allow this range of rotary movements.

About 50% of the flexion-extension movements occur at the occiput and C1 levels, and the balance is evenly distributed between the rest of the cervical vertebrae.

Although lateral bending is a feature of all cervical vertebrae, it does not occur as a pure movement but as a combination with other elements of rotation. When two vertebral bodies are fused, as in Klippel-Feil syndrome, a significant restriction in a specific motion may be caused by blockage in the articulation which provides the greatest amount of movement.

1. *Flexion and extension*:
   The normal range of flexion possible is when the patient can touch his chin to his chest, which can be tested by asking the patient to nod his chest in a forward "yes" movement. The normal range of extension possible is demonstrated when the patient can look directly at the ceiling above him.
2. *Rotation*:
   Ask the patient to shake her head from side to side. The rotations are full when her chin reaches almost to being in line with her shoulders on both sides.
3. *Lateral bending*:
   Ask the patient to try to touch his ears to his shoulders. He should be able to tilt his head approximately 45% toward each shoulder. This movement will be

restricted in cases of enlarged cervical lymph nodes. A similar passive range of movements should be tested when his muscles are fully relaxed. If movements are being tested in a patient with an unstable cervical spine, such as following trauma, avoid testing passive movements in such cases as the neurologic deficit may reoccur or increase.

Neurologic Examination

This is carried out in two stages:

1. Neurologic examination of the intrinsic muscles of the cervical spine and
2. Neurologic examination of the upper extremity by neurologic levels.

Muscle Testing of the Intrinsic Muscles

Flexion:
- *Primary flexors*: Sternocleidomastoids with spinal accessory (spinal XI nerve).
- *Secondary flexors*: Scalenus muscles and prevertebral muscles.

Flexion of the neck is best conducted with the patient seated. The patient's neck is stabilized with one hand and the head is held with the other hand while the patient is asked to bend her neck gently and actively, while gradual resistance is offered against this movement. These findings are then recorded in accordance with the muscle grading chart.

Extension:
- *Primary extensors*: Paravertebral extensor mass (splenius, semispinalis, and capitis) and trapezius with spinal accessory or cranial XI nerve.
- *Secondary extensors*: various small intrinsic neck muscles.
  Stabilize the patient's upper thorax and scapulae by placing a hand to prevent him from substituting trunk extension. Then ask the patient to slowly extend his neck, while applying increased resistance slowly.

Lateral Rotation:
- *Primary rotator*: Sternocleidomastoid with spinal accessory or cranial XI nerve.
- *Secondary rotators*: Small intrinsic neck muscles.
  One sternocleidomastoid contracting alone provides the primary pull for rotation to the side being tested. Ask the patient to say "no" by rotating her head while gradually increasing the resistance offered by the palm of her opposite hand over the side of here mandible.

Lateral Bending:
- *Primary lateral benders*: Scalenus anticus, medius, and posterior.
  Anterior primary divisions of the lower cervical nerves.

- *Secondary lateral benders*: Small intrinsic muscles of the neck.
  Stabilize the shoulder with one hand to prevent shoulder elevation while testing lateral bending, gradually increasing resistance slowly by asking the patient to bend his head laterally.

Examination by Neurologic Levels

Anatomy of the Brachial Plexus

The brachial plexus is formed by eight nerves originating from the first thoracic and lower four cervical levels: namely, C5 to T1. Shortly after emerging from the vertebral bodies and passing between the scalenus anticus and medius, the nerve roots of C5 and C6 join to form the upper trunk.

The nerve root of C7 does not join with any other nerve root but carries on as the middle trunk, while the nerve roots of C8 and T1 join to form the lower trunk. These trunks then pass beneath the clavicle and divide to form cords. These cords are named according to their anatomic relation to the second part of the axillary artery as posterior, lateral, and medial cords of the brachial plexus. The upper trunk (C5 and C6) and the lower trunk (C8 and T1) contribute to the middle trunk (C7) to form the posterior cord. The middle trunk sends a contribution and with C5 and C6 forms the lateral cord. The rest of C8 and T1 forms the medial cord. These branches are called medial, lateral, and posterior depending on their anatomic relation to the second part of the axillary artery. The individual branches from these cords are as follows:

1. From the lateral cord:

   (a) Musculocutaneous nerve.
   (b) Branch to the median nerve.

2. From the medial cord:

   (a) Ulnar nerve.
   (b) Branch to the median nerve.

3. From the posterior cord:

   (a) Axillary nerve.
   (b) Radial nerve.

Sensory Distribution

1. C5 = Lateral arm (axillary nerve)
2. C6 = Lateral forearm, thumb, index, and half of middle finger (sensory branches of the musculocutaneous nerve)

3. C7 = Middle finger
4. C8 = Ring and little fingers, medial forearm (medial antebrachial-cutaneous nerve from the posterior cord)
5. T1 = Medial arm (medial brachial cutaneous nerve from the posterior cord)

Neurologic Level – C5

1. *Muscle testing*:
   The deltoid and biceps are two muscles which are innervated by C5. While the deltoid is solely innervated by C5 (axillary nerve), the biceps has a dual innervation from C5 and C6 (musculocutaneous nerve). The deltoid is a three-part muscle: namely, the anterior, middle, and posterior fibers. The deltoid is tested by resisting the motions of shoulder flexion, abduction, and extension. The biceps acts like a flexor of the shoulder and elbow and also as a supinator of the forearm. The flexion of the elbow can be tested with the forearm supinated as the movement is resisted.
2. *Reflex testing*: Biceps reflex
   The biceps reflex primarily reflects the neurologic integrity of C5. However, the reflex also involves a component of C6.
3. *Sensation testing*:
   Lateral arm – axillary nerve
   The C5 neurologic level is tested by sensations over the lateral arm. This area is useful in diagnosis of injuries to the axillary nerve or general C5 nerve root injury.

Neurologic Level – C6

1. *Muscle testing*:
   Wrist extensors – C6 – radial nerve
   The wrist extensors consist of the following three muscles: (1) the extensor carpi radialis longus – C6, (2) the extensor carpi radialis brevis – C6 and (3) the extensor carpi ulnaris – C7.
   The Biceps C6 (musculocutaneous nerve) can be tested bilaterally.
2. *Reflex testing*:
   Brachioradialis reflex
   This is tested just proximal to the wrist joint when the muscle becomes tendinous just before its insertion to the radius. Also the biceps reflex can be tested here since it is innervated by both C5 and C6.
3. *Sensation Testing*: Lateral forearm – musculocutaneous nerve
   C6 supplies sensation to the lateral forearm, thumb, index and one, and a half portion of the middle finger.

Neurologic Level – C7

1. *Muscle testing*:
   Triceps – C7 – radial nerve
   This muscle can be tested by extension of the elbow with resistance applied to the elbow during extension of the elbow joint.
   Wrist flexors – C7 – median and ulnar nerves
   The wrist flexor group consists mainly of two muscles: (1) the flexor carpi radialis – median nerve and (2) the flexor carpi ulnaris – ulnar nerve. Wrist flexion is tested by asking the patient to flex a closed wrist against resisted flexion.
   Finger extensors – C7 – radial nerve
   Finger extension is done by three muscles: (1) extensor digitorum communis, (2) extensor digiti indicis, and (3) the extensor digiti minimi.
   These can be tested by resisted pressure on the dorsum of the patient's extended fingers.
2. *Reflex testing*:
   Triceps reflex
   This is done by testing the triceps tendon where it crosses the olecranon fossa at the elbow joint.
3. *Sensation testing*: Mainly the middle finger.

Neurologic Level – C8

This level is unique as it does not have any reflex innervations to test, but can be adequately tested by muscle power and sensations.

1. *Muscle testing*: finger flexors
   The two muscles which are finger flexors are (1) the flexor digitorum superficialis (which flexes the PIP joint and is innervated by the median nerve) and (2) the flexor digitorum profundus (which flexes the DIP joint and is innervated by the ulnar nerve on the ulnar side and the median nerve on the radial side). Test the finger flexors by asking the patient to curl or lock her fingers against resisted flexion.
2. *Sensation testing*:
   C8 supplies the ring finger and little fingers of the hand along with the distal half of the ulnar side of the forearm. The ulnar side of the little finger is the ideal site to test for ulnar nerve sensation.

Neurologic Level – T1

This neurologic level is very similar to C8 level with there being no identifiable diagnostic reflex for this level.

Table 8.1 Neurology of the upper extremity

Disc	Root	Reflex	Muscles	Sensation
C4-C5	C5	Biceps reflex	Deltoid and biceps	Lateral arm axillary nerve
C5-C6	C6	Brachioradialis reflex (Biceps reflex)	Wrist extension Biceps	Lateral forearm musculocutaneous nerve
C6-C7	C7	Triceps reflex	Wrist flexors Finger extension Triceps	Middle finger
C7-T1	C8	–	Finger extension	Medial forearm
			Hand intrinsics	Med. ant. brach.
				Cutaneous nerve
T1-T2	T1	–	Hand intrinsics	Medial arm Med. brach. Cutaneous nerve

Table 8.2 The major peripheral nerves

Nerve	Motor test	Sensation test
Radial nerve	Wrist extension	Dorsal web space between thumb and Index finger
	Thumb extension	
Ulnar nerve	Abduction – little finger	Distal ulnar aspect – little finger
Median nerve	Thumb pinch	Distal radial aspect – index finger
	Opposition of thumb	
	Abduction of thumb	
Axillary nerve	Deltoid	Lateral arm – deltoid patch on upper arm
Musculocutaneous nerve	Biceps	Lateral forearm

1. *Muscle testing*:
   The finger abductors are representative of this level. They are innervated by the ulnar nerve and are (1) the dorsal interossei and (2) the abductor digiti quinti. These can be tested by resisted abduction of the fingers together.
2. *Sensation testing*:
   Medial aspect of the arm – medial brachial cutaneous nerve.
   Sensation is tested on the medial side of the upper half of the forearm by the T1 (Tables 8.1 and 8.2).

Special Tests

There are mainly five special tests when dealing with examination of the cervical spine which one has to keep in mind. These are (1) the compression test, (2) the distraction test, (3) the Valsalva test, (4) the swallowing test, and (5) the Adson test.

1. *Compression test*:
   This is done by pressing down on the top of the patient's head. When there is an increase in the pain in the cervical spine or the extremity, that is indicative of one or more of the following: (1) a narrowing of the neural foramen, (2) facet joint pressure, or (3) muscle spasm which is increased by compression.

2. *Distraction test*:
   This test is done by distracting the cervical spine by placing the palm of one hand under the patient's chin and the other hand over the patient's occiput and gradually lifting the head to remove its weight on the neck.

   This test is diagnostic in relieving pain due to neural foramen narrowing and resultant nerve root compression by widening the foramen. It also helps in relieving pressure around facet joint capsules. It may also help in relieving muscle spasm by relaxing the contracted muscles.

3. *The Valsalva test*:
   This is done by asking the patient to hold his breath and bear down on his bowels. This increases any pain due to an increase in the intrathecal pressure because of a space-occupying lesion (herniated disc or tumor) in the cervical spinal canal. The usefulness of this subjective test mainly depends on the response from the patient.

4. *Swallowing test*:
   Pain on swallowing can indicate a pathology of the anterior aspect of the cervical spine such as cervical spine pathology, a bony prominence, or a soft tissue swelling such as a hematoma, infection, or tumor.

5. *The Adson test*:
   This test is done by feeling the radial pulse of the extremity at the wrist. Keeping a hand on the radial pulse, abduct, extend, and externally rotate the arm. Then ask the patient to take a deep breath and turn her head toward the arm being tested. A decrease or obliteration of the radial pulse on this maneuver is indicative of a compression of the subclavian artery, which may be compressed by an extra cervical rib or by a tight scalenus anticus and medius muscles.

   Certain conditions affecting the cervical spine must be kept in mind when examining the cervical spine:

1. *Infantile torticollis*: This condition is also called a congenital muscular torticollis, when one sternomastoid is fibrous and fails to elongate as the child grows, resulting in a deformity. This deformity is very obvious when the child reaches 3–4 years of age, when the affected side of the face is tilted downward with the sternomastoid tendon feeling like a cord and taut, restricting movements away from the deformity. Radiographs are absolutely normal, and the sternomastoid tumor is seen and felt clinically. Conservative treatment is tried at first in the form of stretching, and if this fails, then an open tenotomy is carried out preferably at its upper end, through a small transverse incision. Following this a polythene collar is worn until the child can hold her head correctly.

2. *Prolapsed cervical disc*: The factors responsible for a prolapsed cervical disc are similar to those of a lumbar disc prolase. Here there may be neck signs in the form of pain and stiffness and arm signs affecting the nerve roots. The most

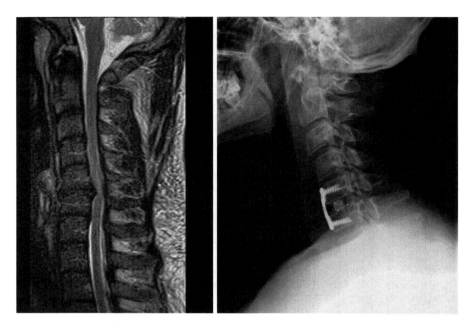

Fig. 8.1 Radiographs showing C56 disc prolapse treated by C56 curettage and fusion (Courtesy Dilip Malhotra, Bahrain)

common areas are the C56 and C67 levels (Fig. 8.1). Radiographs may show an obliteration of the normal cervical lordosis with an early reduction in the disc space level. Careful differential diagnosis must be carried out to rule out cervical rib syndrome, carpal tunnel syndrome, supraspinatus lesions, cervical spine tumors, and infections. Treatment is by rest, traction, and heat with a collar. Very rarely is an operation indicated.

3. *Cervical spondylosis*: This is fairly common after the age of 40 years. It is the most common disorder of the cervical spine when disc material degenerates and extrudes. Radiologically it is seen as lipping of the edges of the vertebral bodies. The patient mainly complains of neck pain with radiation to the occiput or the arms. Treatment is by rest in a soft cervical collar along with cervical traction when necessary. Operative treatment is rarely indicated for this condition, but if it is then a posterior decompressive laminectomy is carried out.

4. *Tuberculosis of the cervical spine*: This is very rarely seen, and the symptoms are variable from neck pain to radicular pain. There is limitation of neck movements along with muscle spasm, and very rarely an abscess may be first found in the retropharyngeal area or just behind the sternomastoid. General antituberculous treatment is initially given, and operative drainage by an anterior incision is advised for drainage of the caseous material, along with interbody fusion using bone grafts from the ribs or the iliac crest.

5. *Cervical rib syndrome*: This is a congenital condition which may be present in various forms. Radiographs are very helpful in diagnosing this condition, as sometimes there may be no neck symptoms and this is accidentally found during other investigations. The patient can have neck or arm symptoms or both. Many conditions closely resemble cervical rib syndrome, such as carpal tunnel syndrome, ulnar tunnel syndrome, Pancoast syndrome, cervical spine lesions or spinal cord lesions, and rotator cuff lesions. Treatment of this condition is mainly conservative in the form of exercises, and very rarely is operative removal indicated – only if the symptoms are very severe with muscular wasting or vascular disturbances.

Chapter 9
Examination of the Lumbar Spine

The brief functions of the lumbar spine are as follows:

1. It transports the cauda equina to the lower limb
2. It provides mobility to the back
3. It provides support to the upper portion of the body and
4. It transmits weight to the pelvis and lower limb.

Inspection

Make sure that the patient takes off all his clothes in order to thoroughly examine the lumbar spine. Take a note of the following:

The condition of the skin, and note any abnormal skin markings – for example, any lipomata, hairy markings, cafe-au-lait spots, any birth markings, or any bony deformity. Small areas of soft masses may be seen in the low back which are indicative of spina bifida, or a dumbbell-shaped lipoma may be seen extending into the cauda equina through a bony defect in the spine. An unusual hairy patch may be seen over certain defects of the spine such as diastematomyelia, or it may be seen with a lipoma referred to as a faun's beard or a mare's tail, which indicates some underlying bony pathology. Skin tags may be seen along with certain areas of dark brown patches in neurofibromatosis, which may impinge on the spinal cord and the spinal nerve roots. Certain birth marks or excessive port wine marks may make one suspicious of some underlying bony pathology, such as spina bifida.

Finally examine the posture in detail. This can be analyzed as follows: With the patient standing, the shoulders should appear square and level. Any inclination or list to one side may indicate sciatic scoliosis in a prolapsed intervertebral disc. Examined sideways, the lumbar spine shows a gentle lordotic curve, which may be exaggerated in a weak anterior abdominal wall. Conversely an extreme sharp deformity or a kyphos may be seen.

K M. Iyer, *Clinical Examination in Orthopedics*,
DOI 10.1007/978-0-85729-971-0_9, © Springer-Verlag London Limited 2012

Palpation

This is best done from behind by placing your fingers on top of the iliac crests and with the thumbs feeling the midline in the back, gradually proceeding upward feeling each bony prominence and each interspace. The spinous processes of L4 and L5 lie above and below the interspace. Proceeding with palpating upward, the spinous processes of the other lumbar vertebrae can be felt. Palpation downward is done by identifying the small spinous process of S2 inferiorly. A visible and palpable step can be felt at the lumbosacral junction indicative of spondylolisthesis.

Proceeding downward, the posterior aspect of the coccyx is clearly felt. This is best palpated by rectal examination, when a painful coccyx may be felt on movement of the mobile coccyx by bimanual examination, suggestive of coccydynia which is fairly common. The examination is completed posteriorly by palpating the posterior superior iliac crests, the greater trochanters, and the ischial tuberosities. The anterior aspect of the lumbar spine is best felt with the patient lying supine with knees bent to relax the abdominal muscles. The umbilicus lies at the level of the L34 interspace, just below which the aorta divides into the common iliac arteries. The anterior aspects of L4 and L5 are palpable below this level to the sacral promontory, which is the prominent portion anteriorly.

After palpating the bony prominences, the soft tissue structures are in five areas:

1. *Midline raphe*: Palpating down the midline over the spinous processes are the supraspinous and interspinous ligaments which may be tender or a defect palpable between the spinous processes. The paraspinal muscles are in three layers of which the superficial layer is easily palpable. This comprises the sacrospinalis system which is made up of spinalis, longissimus, and iliocostalis. These are best palpated by asking the patient to lie prone and lift his head backward. This makes these muscles taut like a cord which may be in spasm and tender.

2. *Iliac crests*: These are palpated throughout their entire length, and the gluteal muscles originate from them.

3. *Posterior superior iliac spines*: These are points of attachment of the sacrotuberous ligaments, and these together with the sacrospinous ligaments bind the sacrum and the ischium to provide for stability of the sacroiliac joint. The sacral triangle is formed by the two posterior superior iliac spines and the top of the gluteal cleft, which may be a spot for tenderness on palpation in low back pain.

4. *Sciatic area*: This nerve is the largest in the body and runs downward posteriorly dividing into two terminal branches – namely, the tibial and peroneal divisions. The sciatic nerve is easily palpated as it passes beneath the piriformis midway between the greater trochanter and the ischial tuberosity.

5. *Anterior abdominal wall and inguinal area*: The anterior abdominal muscles are segmentally innervated from above downward just as the paraspinal muscles. The inguinal area is examined for an abscess within the psoas muscle which can point in this area. Tenderness in this region is usually suggestive of some pathology in the hip joint.

Range of Movements

The lumbar spine has the following movements: flexion, extension, lateral bending, and rotation. These movements are clearly seen, because there are no restraining ribs to limit them.

1. *Flexion*: This is usually tested by asking the patient to bend forward with a straight knee and touch her toes. Inability to do this is measured by the distance from the finger tips to the toes.
2. *Extension*: This is tested by asking the patient to bend gently backward as far as he can.
3. *Lateral bending*: This is not a pure movement but occurs in combination with rotation. Ask the patient to lean to one side as far as she can, by stabilizing the iliac crest with one hand.
4. *Rotation*: This is tested with the patient standing. The iliac crest is stabilized on one side, while the opposite shoulder is being rotated anteriorly or posteriorly.

Neurologic Examination

Each neurologic level is tested for muscles, reflexes, and sensations which receive innervation from that level.

Neurologic Levels T12, L1, L2, and L3

There are no individual reflexes for testing this level.

1. *Muscle testing*: Iliopsoas, which is innervated by T12, L1, L2, and L3.
   This is the main flexor of the hip and is tested by asking the patient to actively raise his thigh while sitting over the edge of the table, with his pelvis stabilized.
2. *Sensation testing*: The sensations to the anterior aspect of the thigh between the inguinal ligament and the knee joint are mainly supplied by the nerves of L1, L2, and L3. These three dermatomes supply this area in an oblique fashion.

Neurologic Levels L2, L3, and L4

1. *Muscle testing*: This is mainly done by testing the quadriceps and the adductors. The quadriceps, which is supplied by the femoral nerve, is tested by asking the patient to extend his knee against resistance while sitting at the edge of the table and with the distal thigh stabilized. The adductors are tested as a group by asking the patient to adduct his legs against resistance, with the patient sitting as when examining the quadriceps.

Neurologic Level L4

1. *Muscle testing*: The tibialis anterior, which is supplied by the deep peroneal nerve.
   This muscle is tested by dorsiflexion and inversion which is resisted on dorsal and medial aspects of the head of the first metatarsal bone.
2. *Reflex testing*: Plantar reflex
   This is a deep tendon reflex supplied by nerves of L2, L3, and L4 – mainly by the L4.
3. *Sensation testing*: This involves the dermatome over the medial side of the leg. The knee represents the dividing line between the L3 and L4 dermatomes. In the leg, the crest of the tibia represents the dividing line between the L4 dermatome on the medial side and the L5 dermatome on the lateral side.

Neurologic Level L5

1. *Muscle testing*: There are three muscles to be tested at this level. The extensor hallucis longus which is supplied by the deep peroneal nerve is tested by placing the thumb on the extensor aspect of the big toe. The patient then dorsiflexes it against resistance. The gluteus medius which is supplied by the superior gluteal nerve is tested by the patient abducting the limb against resistance when lying on her side. The extensor digitorum longus and brevis, which are supplied by the deep peroneal nerve are tested by resisted dorsiflexion of the patient's toes.
2. *Reflex testing*: This is tested by the tibialis posterior reflex which is doubtful and uncertain. This done by tapping on the medial side of the foot just before its insertion into the navicular, holding the foot in dorsiflexion and eversion. This should elicit the plantar inversion response.
3. *Sensation*: This is tested in the dermatome covering the lateral aspect of the leg and the dorsum of the foot.

Neurologic Level S1

1. *Muscle testing*: This is tested in three muscles: The peroneus longus and brevis, which are supplied by the superficial peroneal nerve and are tested by resisting eversion of the plantigrade foot. The gastrocnemius and soleus groups which are supplied by the tibial nerve are tested by the patient resisting plantarflexion of the foot, with the knee straight and kept flexed to 90°. The gluteus maximus which is supplied by the inferior gluteal nerve is tested with the patient lying prone with hips extended and the knees flexed, at which point the tone of the gluteus maximus is palpated.

Table 9.1 Neurology of the lower extremity

Disc	Root	Reflex	Muscles	Sensation
L3-L4	L4	Patellar reflex	Anterior tibialis	Medial leg and Medial foot
L4-L5	L5	None	Extensor hallucis longus	Lateral leg and dorsum of foot
L5-S1	S1	Achilles reflex	Peroneus longus and brevis	Lateral foot

2. *Reflex testing*: Tendoachillis reflex.
   This is a deep tendon reflex which is tested with the patient lying prone. The tendon is tapped while the foot is held in dorsiflexion.
3. *Sensation testing*: The S1 dermatome is tested on the lateral malleolus side and the lateral side and plantar surface of the foot.

Neurologic Level S2, S3, and S4

The S2, S3, and S4 nerves form the principal nerves to the bladder and the intrinsic muscles of the foot. This is best seen as toe deformities, as the bladder cannot be isolated for testing.

There is no deep reflex supplied by S2, S3, and S4.

The perianal sensation is arranged in three concentric rings and tested by a sharp instrument which determines the sensation supplied by S2, S3, and S4/5 dermatomes, with the S4/5 being the innermost ring of supply followed by S3 in the middle and the S2 outermost (Table 9.1).

Superficial Reflexes

There are three main superficial reflexes, which are those of the upper motor neuron. These are mediated through the cerebral cortex or the central nervous system. The patellar tendon and Achilles tendon reflexes are of the lower motor neuron type or deep tendon reflexes requiring tendon stimulation, which are mediated through the anterior horn cell.

1. *Superficial abdominal reflex*: These abdominal muscles are innervated segmentally, the upper muscles from T7 to T10 and the lower muscles from T10 to T11. These muscles are tested by stroking a sharp hammer in each quadrant of the abdominal muscles when their response moves the umbilicus toward the stroked point. This helps in localizing the level of the lesion (a lower motor lesion), by locating the quadrant where the reflex is not seen.
2. *Superficial cremasteric reflex*: This is elicited by stroking the inner side of the upper thigh with a sharp instrument when the scrotal sac on that side is pulled up by the contracting cremaster muscle.
3. *Superficial anal reflex*: This is seen as a contraction of the external and anal sphincter muscles when the perianal skin is stroked.

Pathologic Reflexes

Pathologic reflexes are also superficial reflexes, and their presence indicates an upper motor neuron lesion. There are mainly two tests for these reflexes: namely, the Babinski test and the Oppenheim test.

To elicit the Babinski sign, the test is done by running a sharp instrument along the sole of the foot along the lateral border until the forefoot, to watch for the big toe to extend and the small toe plantar to flex and splay out. A positive Babinski test indicates an upper motor neuron lesion such as an expanding brain tumor. Also note that a positive Babinski test in a newborn is normal and should disappear soon after birth. The Oppenheim test is carried out by running your fingernails along the crest of the tibia. A Babinski-like response is seen, whereas normally there is no response.

Special Tests

There are four sets of special tests:

1. Tests to stretch the spinal cord, cauda equina, or sciatic nerve
2. Tests to increase intrathecal pressure
3. Test to rock the sacroiliac joint and
4. Segmental innervation tests.

Tests to Stretch the Spinal Cord or Sciatic Nerve

There are mainly four of these tests:

The straight leg raising test: This is usually tested to reproduce back and leg pain and is done by gently raising the straight leg as far as possible without causing any pain or discomfort. The normal angle is around 80°. Any decrease in this angle indicates a problem in the sciatic nerve or tightness in the hamstring. When testing the leg, if pain is reproduced in the low back and the opposite leg, then it is a cross leg straight raising test which is positive. When testing this, on dorsiflexion of the foot with the leg raised, there is reproduction of pain along the sciatic nerve.

Well leg straight leg raising test: This test is elicited by raising the patient's unaffected leg, which brings on pain in the opposite side or results in a positive cross leg straight leg raising test.

Hoover test: This is carried out by supporting the extremity under the calcaneus. One can feel the downward pressure on this examining hand as an attempt is made to raise the opposite leg. This mainly helps to differentiate a patient who is malingering, merely stating that he cannot raise his leg.

Kernig test: This is done by placing both the hands behind the patient's back and then flexing his head which reproduces the pain due to a stretch of the spinal cord. The pain may be reproduced in the cervical region, lower back, or even the legs, due to meningeal irritation, nerve root involvement, or irritation of the dural coverings of the nerve root.

Tests to Increase Intrathecal Pressure

There are mainly three tests which demonstrate this effect:

Milgram test: This is performed with the patient lying supine. Ask her to do the straight leg test actively and hold her legs about 2 in. off the table for 30 s without pain. Being able to hold the legs in this position will rule out any intrathecal pressure, while reproduction of pain will indicate intrathecal pathology or pressure.

Naffziger's test: This is tested by gently compressing both the jugular veins until the patient's face begins to flush. Then ask the patient to cough. If there is pain, it indicates increased intrathecal pressure.

Valsalva maneuver: This test is carried out by asking the patient to bear down on his bowels. An increase in pain is indicative of increased intrathecal pressure.

Tests to Rock the Sacroiliac Joint

There are three main tests for this:

Pelvic rock test: With the patient lying supine, try compressing the pelvis by holding the iliac crests. Pain is indicative of some sacroiliac pathology.

Gaenslen's test: This is test is carried out by the patient lying supine on the table with both his legs folded up toward his chest. The patient is shifted to the side of the table with one leg being dropped to the table, while the other is held flexed as before. Pain in the unsupported limb may indicate some sacroiliac pathology.

Patrick or Fabere test: This test is done with the patient lying supine. The involved foot is placed on the opposite knee. The affected side is stabilized on the iliac crest while downward pressure is applied on the bent knee to stress the sacroiliac joint. If pain is elicited, that indicates pathology of the sacroiliac joint.

Neurologic Segmental Innervation Test

Beevor's sign: The rectus abdominis is segmentally innervated by the anterior primary division of T5 to T12. When the patient tries to do a quarter sit-up with his arms across his chest, the umbilicus does not move at all. The umbilicus is drawn toward the stronger side. This sign is frequently positive in patients having poliomyelitis or a meningomyelocele.

Examination of Related Areas

Most importantly, it is imperative to perform a rectal examination in all male patients and a pelvic examination in all female patients.

Certain specific conditions must be borne in mind when examining the thoracolumbar spine:

1. *Tuberculosis of the spine*: Spinal tuberculosis is fairly common and also the most dangerous form of tuberculosis. It usually starts in the body of one vertebra, which gets squashed thereby affecting the vertebra above and below. This squeezes out caseous material to gradually involve the spinal cord or escape into the soft tissues as a cold abscess. With time, healing occurs by a solid bony fusion with angulation resulting in a kyphotic deformity. Treatment is usually started by antituberculous drugs along with bed rest on a plaster bed or in a brace or back support. Surgical operative treatment is undertaken when the general condition permits, anteriorly by evacuation of the abscess, caseous bone, and curettage, and the cavity is plugged with iliac bone grafts. Serial follow-ups are made to keep in mind the two most important complications – namely, paraplegia and a flare-up of the disease. The patient may present with paraplegia, at which point an aggressive method of treatment by a complete, thorough decompression is undertaken.

2. *Scoliosis*: Deviation of the spine to one side when seen from behind is called scoliosis. There are two main forms:

   (a) *Mobile scoliosis*: Here the vertebrae are rotated, which is transient and never develops into the fixed type of scoliosis. There are three main subvarieties of mobile scoliosis: (i) the postural variety is very common in adolescent girls and the curvature is usually to the left side (Fig. 9.1). The spine straightens out when the child bends forward; (ii) compensatory mobile scoliosis which is commonly seen in limb length inequality. Here the curve disappears when the child sits; (iii) sciatic mobile scoliosis, in which there is a lateral tilt to one side which usually accompanies a slipped disc.

   (b) *Fixed scoliosis*: This is a structural variety which is always accompanied by rotation of the vertebrae. This deformity keeps on growing until skeletal spinal maturity, as noticed by the Risser's sign of the iliac apophyses on radiographs. Various varieties of fixed scoliosis are seen such as idiopathic, congenital, paralytic, neurofibromatosis, and in syringomyelia. The presenting complaint is deformity, but combined curves above and below may pass unnoticed. Usually the patient is a young adolescent girl who presents with a rib hump due to vertebral rotation. Radiologic measurements are then carried out on full-length films to get the exact angle of curvature between unwedged discs at the end of the primary curve. Treatment is usually conservative combined with follow-up

Fig. 9.1 Full-length weight-bearing anteroposterior radiograph of a 15-year-old girl during school screening (Courtesy Dushyant Thakkar, London, UK)

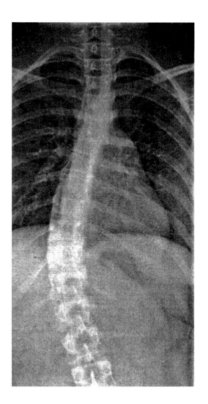

every 3 months. Conservative treatment is by supports which are useful in certain cases. Three kinds are available (i) a distraction plaster jacket which is applied on a Risser jacket, (ii) a Milwaukee brace with adjustable steel supports and (iii) a Boston brace which extends from the pelvis to the thoracic cage. Operative treatment is indicated for curves over 70°. Operative treatment is also indicated in younger patients, those with greater curves or paralytic curves, and in patients with neurofibromatosis. A preoperative myelogram is essential to exclude diastematomyelia in congenital scoliosis. Operative treatment mainly involves correction and fusion of the entire primary curve.

3. *Kyphosis*:

   These are classified into three types: namely,

   (a) *Mobile kyphosis*, which may be (i) postural such as in patients with flat feet or (ii) based on muscular weakness as seen in poliomyelitis or muscular dystrophies or (iii) compensatory to lumbar lordosis.

   (b) *Fixed kyphosis*: This is usually seen in (i) Scheuermann's disease, (ii) ankylosing spondylitis, or (iii) senile kyphosis.

   (c) *Angular kyphosis or kyphos*: This is usually a fixed variety and forward angulation may be (i) congenital, (ii) tuberculous, or (iii) following a fracture (Fig. 9.2) or (iv) due to Calve's disease.

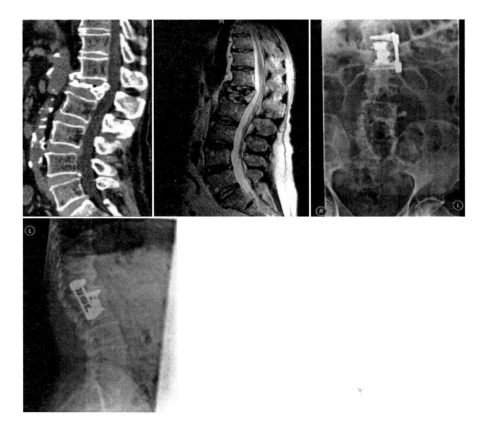

Fig. 9.2 Magnetic resonance imaging showing an unstable fracture of L1 with an internal gibbus, treated by internal fixation with correction of the internal gibbus (Courtesy Dushyant H. Thakkar, London, UK)

4. *Lumbar disc prolapse*: The nucleus pulposus is normally under tension and is surrounded by the fibrous annulus which is held in place by ligaments. Displacement occurs due to (a) prolapse of the disc substance into the vertebral canal, (b) extrusion around the periphery as seen in spondylosis or (c) protrusion into the vertebral bodies as seen in Scheuermann's resulting in Schmorl's nodes.

   With age as the disc degenerates and loses elasticity, partly because of the physiochemical changes in its collagen fibers and partly because of a decrease in its fluid content, the weakened disc cannot resist the body weight and hence bulges (Fig. 9.3). This prolapsed disc may press on the dura or on the nerve roots. The patient is usually an adult, and the first attack is usually sudden while bending forward. There may be associated signs in the legs due to root pressure. Radiographs of the lumbar spine are essential. These may be helpful in showing a decreased disc space. The precise location of the disc prolapsed is best seen on myelography.

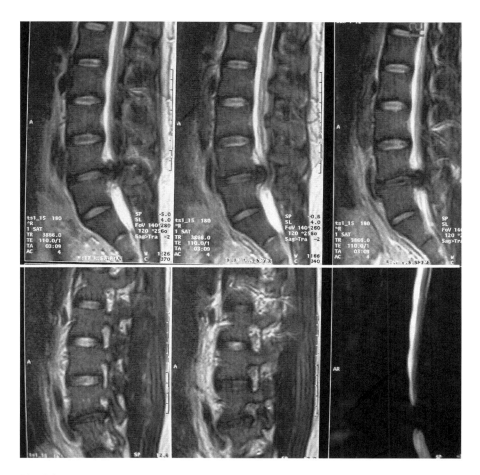

Fig. 9.3 Myelogram showing the exact location of a disc prolapse (Courtesy Dilip Malhotra, Bahrain)

Certain disorders must be excluded in a differential diagnosis such as tuberculosis, osteomyelitis, discitis, ankylosing spondylitis (Fig. 9.4), sacroiliac disease, or tumors. Treatment of this condition mainly involves bed rest along with traction, analgesics, lumbosacral corset, and gradually gentle exercises to strengthen the back muscles. Very rarely is manipulation helpful, and in some cases an epidural injection of steroids with lignocaine is helpful to reduce the acute pain. Should these methods fail to improve the condition, then an operative intervention in the form of a laminectomy with removal of the offending disc is considered.

5. Lumbar spondylosis with resultant disc degeneration results in a constant backache. This is treated by bed rest, analgesics, heat, and a lumbar corset. Rarely is surgery in the form of a spinal fusion indicated in these cases.

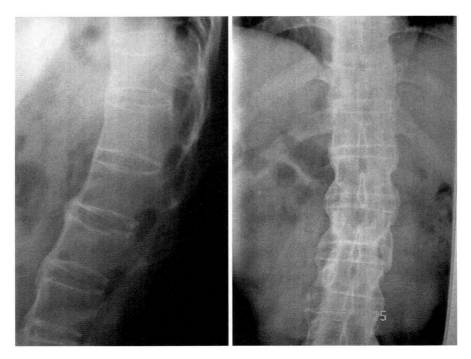

Fig. 9.4 Radiographs of the lumbar spine, showing ankylosing spondylitis (Courtesy Dilip Malhotra, Bahrain)

6. *Spinal stenosis*: Here the spinal canal is congenitally small, and symptoms are aggravated by a disc prolapse or any intraspinal pathology (Fig. 9.5). It is usually relieved by a decompressive laminectomy.

7. *Spondylolisthesis*: This involves a forward shift of the spine and is usually seen between L4 and L5 or between L5 and the sacrum (Fig. 9.6).

   Three main types are recognized: namely (a) dysplastic, when the sacral facets are congenitally defective, (b) degenerative changes are seen in the facet joints which allow a forward slip and (c) the isthmic when the lamina is in two pieces along with a gap in the pars interarticularis. This may be seen accidentally during routine radiographic examination, and oblique views show the gap extremely clearly. Treatment usually consists of conservative treatment in the form of a corset along with graduated exercises. Should they not be helpful, then operative treatment in the form of a posterolateral fusion or an anterior fusion is considered.

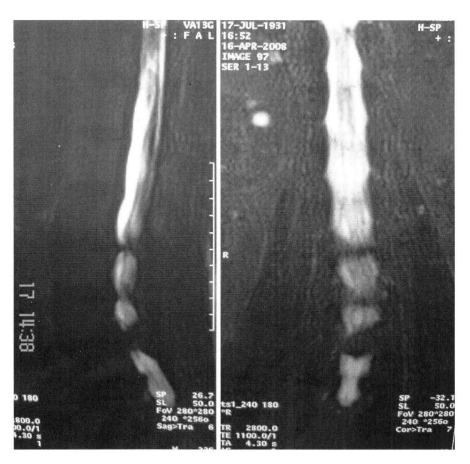

Fig. 9.5 An magnetic resonance imaging myelogram showing multilevel spinal stenosis (Courtesy Dilip Malhotra, Bahrain)

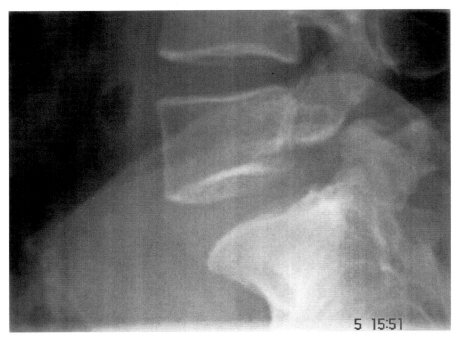

Fig. 9.6 Radiograph showing spondylolisthesis of L5 over S1 (Courtesy Dilip Malhotra, Bahrain)

Chapter 10
Examination of the Temporomandibular Joint

This is the most used joint in the body, and it performs various functions such as chewing, talking, swallowing, yawning, and snoring. Examination of this joint is completed with inspection, palpation, range of movements, and neurologic examination and a special test for this joint.

Inspection

It is located just anterior to the external auditory meatus and can be seen in movements when the mandible is in motion. It has mainly two phases of joint motion: namely (1) a swing phase when it is in motion and (2) a stance phase when the mouth is closed. In the swing phase, the rhythm of opening and closing the jaw is smooth, regular, and in the midline with the teeth coming together and separating easily. In the stance phase, the jaw is in the midline, and the teeth are closed symmetrically in the midline. The temporomandibular joint is not a true weight-bearing joint since the weight is transmitted through the teeth to the maxilla, but it is often converted into one giving pain and headache when a patient with poor dentition is placed in cervical traction.

The joint moves by a hinge and glide movement within the glenoid fossa and finally glides forward to rest on the eminentia. Like other joints having more than one type of movement, there is an articular disc or the meniscus which divides the joint into two halves – namely, the upper half for hinge movement and the lower part which is used for gliding. This is carried out by the dual heads of the external pterygoid muscles acting synchronously, with one head pulling the meniscus forward while the other opens the joint.

Palpation

This is done by placing the index finger in the patient's external auditory canal while asking the patient to open and close his mouth gently. The movement of the mandibular condyle is felt beneath the tip of the examining finger. This movement is smooth and bilaterally symmetrical, and any crepitus or clicking that is heard may be suggestive of a tear in the meniscus of the temporomandibular joint. When the patient opens his mouth wide open, both the temporomandibular joints may dislocate anteriorly with a clunk. Such dislocations may cause soft tissue damage to the joint capsule, and the meniscus may also tear, resulting in stretching of the external pterygoid muscle giving rise to muscular spasms. Asymmetrical dentition may cause a palpable click in the external auditory canal, and a constant grinding or clicking (bruxism) may overload the joint giving rise to symptoms.

The external pterygoid muscle is palpated for spasm and tenderness by placing the index finger between the buccal mucosa and the superior gum and pointing the tip of the index finger posteriorly past the last upper molar toward the neck of the mandible. This muscle can be felt as a tight cord with pain and tenderness when the patient opens and closes his mouth.

Range of Motion

Ask the patient to open her mouth, and she should be able to do this movement to accommodate three fingers between her incisor teeth. The mandible should also be able to glide forward to protrude such that the bottom teeth can be placed in front of the top teeth. These movements can be tested passively if the patient is unable to actively test them, and even this may be limited in cases of muscle spasm, rheumatoid arthritis, or certain congenital bony anomalies or bony ankylosis of the temporomandibular joint.

Neurologic Examination

Muscle Testing

This is tested by opening the mouth and closing the mouth.

Opening the mouth: The primary opener is the external pterygoid muscle, which is supplied by the pterygoid branch of the mandibular division of the trigeminal nerve. The secondary openers are the hyoid muscles and gravity. These can be tested by placing the hand under the jaw against resistance while the patient attempts to open the mouth. Normally, it should be possible to open the mouth against maximum resistance.

   Closing the mouth: The primary closers are the masseters and the temporalis muscles, which are both supplied by the trigeminal nerve. The secondary closer is the internal pterygoid muscle. This can be tested by forcing the closed mouth into an open position with the hand.

Reflex Testing: Jaw Reflex

This reflex is tested with a reflex hammer, holding a finger over the mental area of the chin while the jaw is slightly open. The reflex will close the mouth. It may be diminished or absent due to pathology along the trigeminal nerve or may be exaggerated in an upper motor lesion.

Special Test for the Temporomandibular Joint

Chvostek test: This tests the seventh (facial) cranial nerve and is done by tapping the parotid gland overlying the masseter muscle. A facial contraction in the form of a twitch occurs only if the blood calcium is low.

Chapter 11
Examination of Gait

Kinesiology, as well as motion picture photography of human subjects at rest and in motion, is required for a detailed study and application of the knowledge of human gait. For an average clinician, these studies are neither easily available nor understandable. With these facts in mind, this chapter is entirely devoted to human gait as a clinician should know it.

"Gait" is defined as the rhythmic movements of the joints of the lower extremity, resulting in forward propagation of the body. Thus it differs from spot March – as in exercises – where rhythm is essential, but there is no forward propagation.

Human gait is a *biped gait,* whereas animal gait is *quadruped.*[1] In quadrupeds, the hind limbs are used for propulsion and the fore limbs are meant for restriction. The extension of the hind limbs imparts momentum, and the fore limbs restrict this momentum when they touch the ground. In human beings, each leg performs these functions alternately. Thus human gait may be described as *alternate bipedalism.* It is essentially a "heel–toe" gait, with the heel touching the ground first, followed by the toes, and, again, the heel leaving the ground before the toes.

Human gait is a *biphasic gait* wherein there is a *stance phase* and a *swing phase.* In the stance phase, both feet are on the ground, and in the swing phase, alternate lower limbs swing forward. Tension in the hamstring muscles restricts the extent of the swing, and the heel strike restricts forward momentum. Thus the stance phase starts at *heel strike,* and lasts through *foot flat* and *toes strike* before ending after *toe rise* when the swing phase starts. In the complete stance both feet are flat on ground.

When we look at various people walking, each of them seems to have a gait that is different from the others, yet all of them are deemed to have a normal gait. It must, however, be understood that the visible differences among the gaits is essentially in movement, sway or attitude of torsos, or gestures by the movement of the upper limbs. *Normal gait,* therefore, is rhythmic movement of the lower limbs.

---

[1] Exceptions include frogs and toads, who have biped gait, though it is unlike human gait.

Fig. 11.1 Trendelenburg's
test positive (**a**), and
negative (**b**)

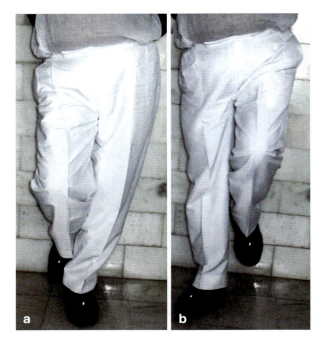

Now, let us consider the movements of the joints of the lower extremity in a normal gait. In the swing phase, there is obviously flexion of the hip joint. When one
stands on one leg, the unsupported pelvis would be expected to fall because of gravity. However, this does not happen; the unsupported pelvis is actually elevated by
the abductor muscles of the supported limb, which are abducting the supported hip.
This is demonstrated by the rise of the anterior superior iliac spine or of the gluteal
crease on the unsupported side. This is Trendelenburg's test for assessing hip
stability (Fig. 11.1).

At every swing, there is abduction of the opposite hip; to neutralize this, during
the swing phase, there is an adduction of the ipsilateral hip. This movement occurs
even if the adductor muscles are paralyzed, because the hip joint is of the ball and
socket variety, and the limb adducts due to gravity. Again, in the swing phase, the
pelvis is oblique in the sagittal plane; the ipsilateral half being anterior to the con-
tralateral half, resulting in the internal rotation of the supported hip. To neutralize
this, there is an external rotation of the ipsilateral hip. To summarize: there is flexion, adduction, and external rotation of the ipsilateral hip during the swing phase.

During the swing phase, after initial flexion, there is gradual extension of the
knee joint until it is fully extended at heel strike. This initial flexion is necessary to
clear the ground, and is secondary to the plantar flexion at the ankle.

At the onset of the swing phase, there is plantar flexion of the ankle joint, resulting in push-off. Later on, there is dorsiflexion of the ankle to help clear the ground.
The swing phase ends upon heel strike.

Fig. 11.2 Abnormal gaits

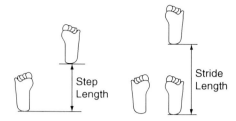

Step Length

Stride Length

To summarize: during swing phase, there is

Flexion, adduction, and external rotation of the hip,
After initial flexion, extension of the knee and
After initial plantar flexion, dorsiflexion of the ankle.

These are the movements in the lower limb that characterize normal gait. Any variation from these will result in an abnormal gait. A minor variation may be termed a limp. A major deviation may result in a visible body shift – i.e., a lurch – to neutralize various other forces.

Step length is the distance between the right and left heels when a step is taken. It corresponds to the length of the foot and about an additional 25 cm. In an average adult, this works out to between 45 and 50 cm. Stride length is the distance covered by the same heel after a stride. It varies according to the length of the lower limb and consequently depends on the height of the individual. A tall person covers more ground than a short person in a given period of time. Each individual usually takes a certain number of steps per minute. This is known as his/her "cadence," and varies with individuals. An altered cadence cannot be sustained for a long time as it causes fatigue, and one may not be able to walk continuously faster or slower than one's own style without becoming tired. There is a thin margin of difference between a fast walk and a slow run. During a walk, there is always a stage when both feet are on the ground – this is called the "stance." During a run, there is always a phase when both feet are off the ground. Thus feet should be closely watched to differentiate between these two (Fig. 11.2).

Now we look at some abnormal gaits.

Antalgic gait: Any gait that relieves pain is known as an antalgic gait. Its visual characteristics cannot be described as they depend upon the source of the pain and the manner of obtaining relief from it.

High stepping gait: As mentioned earlier, there is dorsiflexion of the ankle joint during the swing phase. If there is loss of dorsiflexion due to a plantar flexion deformity or loss of muscle power, there will be difficulty in getting clear of the ground during the swing. To avoid this, one has to flex one's hip more than usual, thus raising the knee and the foot off the ground. This gait is common in foot drop due to muscle paralysis (Fig. 11.3).

Stamping gait: In affections of the posterior column of the spinal cord, there is loss of joint and vibration sense. Thus one is not able to perceive the distance of the

Fig. 11.3 High step with foot drop

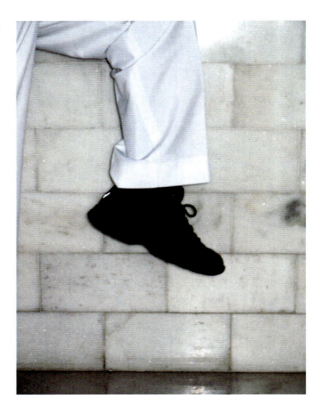

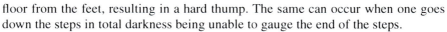

Fig. 11.4 Broad-based gait

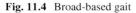

floor from the feet, resulting in a hard thump. The same can occur when one goes down the steps in total darkness being unable to gauge the end of the steps.

Broad-based gait: In earlier times on boats at sea, there was always a sense of instability due the swaying and tossing of the boat when the sea was rough. To overcome this and to prevent accidental falls, sailors would walk with their feet fairly wide apart (Fig. 11.4). This served to keep the center of gravity within the base and helped avoid falls. This habit at sea also manifested itself when the sailors walked on land. Such a gait is rarely seen in the present environment because of stabilizers in modern boats.

Hemiplegic gait: In ambulatory hemiplegic patients there is rigidity in the lower limb muscles because of an upper motor neuron lesion (Fig. 11.5). Due to this, extension at the knee and plantar flexion at the ankle prevail. As stated earlier,

Fig. 11.5 Hemiplegic gait

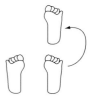

Fig. 11.6 Scissors gait

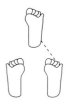

during the swing phase, there is flexion at the knee and dorsiflexion at the ankle. The swing of lower limb in hemiplegic patients, therefore, becomes difficult. In such cases, there is circumduction of the limb at the hip while swinging the limb to achieve forward propulsion.

Scissors gait: In lesions resulting in spastic paraparesis, each lower limb crosses in front of the other lower limb, due to a marked adduction spasm as is commonly seen in cerebral palsy patients (Fig. 11.6).

Ataxic gait: In cerebellar lesions there is loss of a sense of balance. Such loss prevents righting reflexes from coming into play. The patient is unable to balance himself and sways in various directions during ambulation.

Trendelenburg's gait: In cases of malunited or ununited fractures of the neck of the femur, dislocations or subluxations of the hip joint, coax vara, and paralysis of hip abductors, there is a loss of hip stability due to an inefficient abductor lever. As a result of this, there is a drooping of the opposite half of the pelvis when the weight is borne on the affected limb. This will render ground clearance by the opposite limb difficult. To overcome this problem, when the weight is borne on the affected side, the body or torso swings on the same side and the help of the quadratus lumborum muscle is made use of to lift the opposite half of the pelvis. Thus the pelvis dips on the opposite side and the trunk swings on the same side. This is also known as the "gluteus medius gait."

If such lesions are bilateral, the same sequence occurs on both sides and the "waddling gait" results. The same type of gait is present in osteomalacic patients due to a muscle weakness secondary to calcium deficiency.

Short limb gait: For obvious reasons, the pelvis dips and the trunk swings on the same side when weight is borne on the affected side. If there is an associated hip instability, the gluteus medius gait prevails.

Gluteus maximus gait: In paralysis of the gluteus maximus muscle, it is not possible to extend the supported hip in the swing phase. This is overcome by a backward lurch of the trunk.

Fig. 11.7 In-toeing

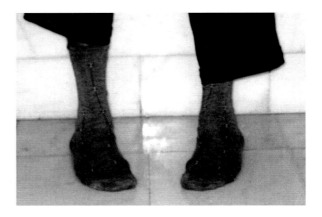

In-toeing gait: In cases of increased anteversion of the femoral neck, there is internal rotation of the hip joint to contain the femoral head in the acetabular cavity. This results in an internal rotation of the whole limb as noted by inward pointing toes. Such in-toeing may persist (Fig. 11.7), or compensatory changes may occur to offset this disability. There is external torsion of the tibia, and toes point forward. However, persistent femoral torsion is evident by both patellae pointing inward rather than forward – this is referred to as "kissing patellae." At the time of correcting this deformity, care should be taken to note if corrective changes have occurred. If so, corrective derotation osteotomy of both the femur and the tibia will be necessary. If both bones are not attended to, out-toeing will result – a Charlie Chaplin type of gait.

Shuffling gait: In this type of gait, slow and short steps are taken. This can be due to arthrosis of the hips and spine, which prevents any compensatory mechanisms to overcome loss of movements. Such a gait can also result from marked rigidity as in Parkinson's disease. Thus, there may be an arthritic shuffle or a parkinsonian shuffle.

Stiff knee gait: When a person has a loss of movements at the knee joint, the gait looks like that of a German soldier marching.

Flexed knee gait: The gait is a short limb gait with the knee flexed.

Hand-to-knee gait: In a two-leg stance, the line of gravity passes from posterior to the hip, anterior to the knee, and through the ankle joint. When there is a quadriceps deficiency, one would expect the knee to buckle down during the stance phase. However, this does not happen, because gravity does not cause knee flexion. As a corollary to this, it can be stated that quadriceps functional deficiency will not affect ambulation. As a matter of fact, ambulation is possible with accessory muscles.

In the one-leg stance with the affected limb in front, there is always the possibility of the knee buckling down when the opposite limb starts swinging because the body mass is largely posterior. If the affected limb is rotated externally at the hip, knee flexion due to gravity cannot occur because it would cause knee abduction, which is not possible at that joint. Thus in extensor weakness at the knee there will

Fig. 11.8 Hand-to-knee gait

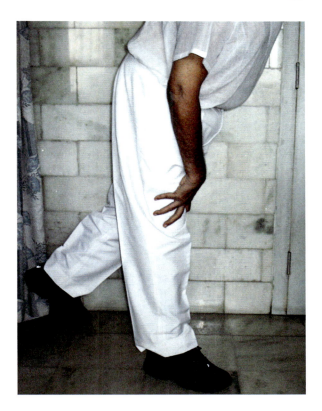

be an external rotation gait. If there is paralysis of the quadriceps femoris muscle, other muscles are used to prevent buckling down. Extensors of the hip joint move the femur backward. The soleus muscle moves the tibia backward when the foot is on the ground. Thus the gluteus acting from above and the soleus acting from below move the femur and the tibia, respectively, backward to cause hyperextension at the knee to prevent buckling down. Hyperextension gait then results.

When either or neither of these muscles is functioning well, the patient bodily pushes the lower end of the femur backward with his hand to achieve hyperextension. This results in the hand-to-knee gait (Fig. 11.8).

Calcaneus gait: Just before the limb swing, there is a push-off at the ankle joint by plantar flexion (Fig. 11.9). This push-off is absent in paralysis or rupture of the tendoachillis. The weight is largely borne by the heel, and there is a widening and thickening of the heel. The gait is slower and without heel push-off; the foot is flat on the ground.

Flat foot gait: When there is affection of the arches of the foot, the foot is flat on the ground and there is no spring in the gait. The speed is slower and occasionally there is pain.

Fig. 11.9 Calcaneus gait

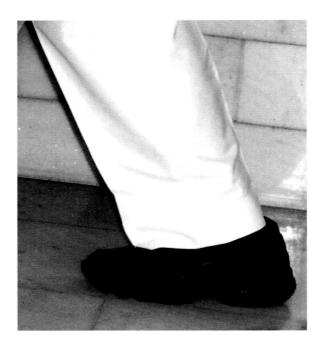

At times one comes across a gait which looks abnormal but is really not so because one is observing the body and not the lower limbs.

In cases with a rigid lumbar spine, the gait resembles that of the Lord Mayor of London marching on a ceremonial occasion.
In tuberculosis of the dorsal spine, the patient often walks with hands on the thighs to off-load his/her body weight and to bypass the affected spine.
In tuberculosis of the cervical spine, the patient holds his head and neck in his hands to bypass the affected spine.

There are variations of normal gait, which may look abnormal, but are not so.
Athlete's gait: One might notice a difference in the gait of players before and after a game. When they are returning at the end of a game, their attitude shows crouching. This attitude is adopted to keep their center of gravity as low as possible. It prevents fatigue.
Exaggeration of normal oscillations: As stated earlier, there is forward and side-ward swing of the body during walking. This swing keeps the center of gravity shifting within the body. Such a shift results in oscillations of the body. Exaggeration of these oscillations is often resorted to artificially to draw attention.
Mourner's gait: At a solemn occasion like a funeral, there are mourners of various heights walking at different speeds. However, the whole crowd moves together, and none become separated from the rest. One may expect a short person to walk faster by increasing cadence. This will cause fatigue and hence is not practical. One

Fig. 11.10 Mourner's gait

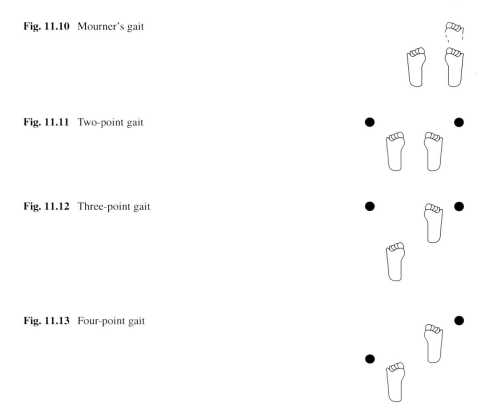

Fig. 11.11 Two-point gait

Fig. 11.12 Three-point gait

Fig. 11.13 Four-point gait

may expect a tall person to walk slower by altering his or her cadence. Again, this is not practical. Altered cadence cannot be sustained for a long time, as it will produce fatigue. To maintain a semblance of order, a tall person shortens his step length without altering his cadence. He takes a forward stride but brings his foot slightly back to shorten his step length (Fig. 11.10). There is a lot of mechanical disadvantage and loss of energy during this gait. It is, however, necessary in paying respect to a departed soul and on solemn occasions.

Crutch gait: When using crutches, we need to consider crutches and legs as four points. Either crutches move together or legs move together. Also there are occasions when all of these four points move separately.

Two-point gait: When a double amputee walks with crutches there is a two-point gait. Crutches are put forward and then swinging moves the body forward (Fig. 11.11). One may swing up to the crutches or swing through them – in a "swing-to" or "swing-through" gait.

Three-point gait: When weight is allowed only on one leg, crutches are put forward and the limb follows with the other limb off the ground. This is the three-point gait (Fig. 11.12). It could also be a swing-to or swing-through gait.

Four-point gait: When limbs are allowed to bear weight but are not strong enough to do so unaided, a pair of crutches is used for ambulation. Crutches and legs are alternately put forward singly to achieve the four-point gait (Fig. 11.13).

Knowledge of gait helps one to arrive at a diagnosis and to assess the degree of disability before a detailed examination is done. The patient must be examined by gait inspection before palpation, motion estimation, and measurements are undertaken and the rest of the body is examined.

Acknowledgments   I greatly appreciate the help of my son Mr. Niraj L. Vora, M.S. (Orth), M.R.C.S. (Edin), Joint Replacement Surgeon, Kokilaben Dhirubhai Ambani Hospital, Mumbai, for taking all of the photographs and drawing the diagrams used in this chapter.

L.N. Vora, M.S. (Bom.), F.C.P.S. (Bom.), F.R.C.S. (Eng.), M.Ch.Orth. (L'Pool)
Hon. Orthopaedic Surgeon, Sir. H.N. Hospital, Mumbai.

Hon. Prof. Of Orthopaedics (Retd.) Seth G.S. Medical College, Mumbai.

Hon. Orthopaedic Surgeon (Retd.) K.E.M. Hospital, Mumbai.

Index